A Stranger In Our House

A Stranger In Our House

A Family Faces Breast Cancer

By Chris Grayson
with Fred Hill

Writer's Showcase
San Jose New York Lincoln Shanghai

A Stranger In Our House
A Family Faces Breast Cancer

Writer's Showcase
an imprint of iUniverse, Inc.

For information address:
iUniverse, Inc.
5220 S. 16th St., Suite 200
Lincoln, NE 68512
www.iuniverse.com

Please consult your doctor to determine your best means on treatment.

ISBN: 0-595-22630-2

Printed in the United States of America

To my loving wife, Karen

Thank you for allowing me to share our story in this book. Even though I've shared some of your most private moments in these pages, it has been my therapy through these tough times.

**To our children
Michael, Michelle and Stephen**

Thanks for being so supportive and understanding. Being young like you are it is hard to understand some of the things we did during the summer and fall of 2000. I hope when you read this book you will understand why we did what we did.

I would like to thank everyone who helped us during this most difficult time of our life. My thanks are not limited to the people listed on this page. But everyone listed here played a roll in our recovery and made our burdens lighter to bear. We could never repay you for your help. We will never forget what you've done for us.

James and Elsa Grayson
Jeff and Vickie Grayson
Paul and JoLynn Grayson
Wesley and Sandra Beal
Charles and Kay Beal
Larry and Janet Bradshaw
Becky Zimmerman
Dewey and Sally Parker
Billy and Marianne Smith
Clyde and Pauline Zimmerman
Ronda Hostetler
Angela Martin
Mike Sandifar
Mark And LaDonna Johnson
Richard & Cheryl Gilbert
Rev. James Cash and Esther
Amy Bousquet
Northaven Elementary School Staff

Fred,

My sincere thanks for help in writing this book. I would have never thought I could of written this book without you help. I'm sure there are a few professors in my past that never thought I could have accomplished this either.

Your help in getting me to fully express our story in words is most appreciated. You have a talent I only wish I had. I can just see your father sitting in front of his television set watching endless hours of basketball, and your mother right beside him reading a book. I think she would of appreciated our effort. They were great neighbors to have and our lives were blessed by having them as neighbors in the last years of their life.

As you and Barbara prepare to move to Florida I wish you the best. As you spend time watching your neighbors yachts go by, please remember, if the excitement is too much for you to handle, you can always return for a visit to Charlestown.

Thank you so much,

Chris

I would also like to thank the American Cancer Society for providing me with useful information through their 1-800 For Cancer telephone number. They provided me with two pamphlets titled "Understanding Breast Cancer Treatment" A Guide For Patients and "What You Need To Know About Breast Cancer" both by the National Institute of Health and the National Cancer Institute.

I used information from these pamphlets in this book and during our cancer treatment. They were welcomed sources of information that was easily read and understood. My thanks to them for the service they provide to people in need such as Karen and I.

INTRODUCTION:
The Emotional Roadmap

by Fred Hill

One slings around a lot of sloppy emotions during a family crisis. Tears fly, rages erupt all too easily…none of us are at our best during such times. The author of this book, a funeral director and the partner in his wife's challenge against breast cancer knows this all too well. So do I. I share a sleepy little block in Charlestown, Indiana with the Grayson Funeral Home, and ushered both of my parents through its doors while the Grayson family fought their own battles. My wife and I discovered the difficulties and unexpected rewards of acting as caregivers during my parents' last days. Our experience was recorded in a book, Outrunning Your Shadow: Caring for Dying Parents.

Somewhere in my book (still selling at **www.fredhill.net** or at typical Internet outlets, in case you were wondering) I claimed that the loss of one's parents represents the biggest crisis in most of our lives. A reviewer challenged this statement, citing her own battle to care for her spouse. The marriage cut short, the love so soon lost, the loneliness ahead…This, she said is life's greatest drama.

Ever defensive, I reassured myself that the numbers were on my side. More than half of us will never lose our partner, because we either choose to live without one or we die first. The loss of a child, certainly more painful by any measure, is gratefully spared many parents. My statement remained valid in my mind. Yet the reviewer had made an important point: her ordeal must have been so much worse than mine.

As if to teach me this lesson, my neighbor Chris Grayson consulted me with the manuscript of a book he was working on. "You're supposed to know about words and books and things like that. Tell me what you think about this." He dropped it off to me with a careless gesture, like a student turning in his last minute term paper. Body language suggested that it was a silly little writing assignment. But I could tell it meant a lot more to him.

Well, this is what I think, Chris. I think the Grayson's story is helpful, moving, and important. I think their ordeal can help prepare others for the stresses and shocks of an all-too-common challenge in our fragile lives. I think Chris captured the story with frankness and humility, as well as some simple straightforward Hoosier charm. He also sketched a portrait of Karen Grayson that is real and sympathetic, vulnerable and courageous. It is a memorable portrayal of a woman who has demonstrated the heroism necessary to stare defiantly down the throat of an attaching intruder.

The pain of this story belongs to Karen and Chris Grayson, their children and friends, and the many millions who have faced or are facing breast cancer. The love in this story belongs to Chris and Karen, who clung to each other and shared their strength while crashing through uncharted waters. The words of this story belong to Chris, I can only take cosmetic credit for this fine book.

But I have learned from their story of love and fear, and I hope you will too. They decided to share this hard time in their lives to help others. This book maps out their emotional trek through denial and obsession, guilt and depression, toward a deeper love and richer life. It offers information on breast cancer and its treatment, with a special focus on the impact such a diagnosis can have on husband and family. The author urges his readers to take preventative steps, to arm themselves with the knowledge and assert their roles in their own medical care. And he cries out for a more supportive "hospital policy" to afford the spouse a rightful role in the care of the patient.

Above all, the book discusses breast cancer with an unflinching honesty. It's a topic too important to ignore, and too painful to postpone until it becomes urgent in your life.

If you ever find yourself in Charlestown, Indiana check your map to make sure you haven't made a mistake. If not proceed to High Street and drop by the Grayson Funeral Home. You'll find that Chris in person distinctly resembles Chris in print. Life is too precious in small-town Indiana to waste time putting on any airs. There's always after school activities to attend, covered-dish church socials to organize, friends in need to counsel and comfort. The Graysons keep so busy with all these activities that they asked me to do the detail work on this book. These days we call it "having a life," and Chris and Karen wouldn't trade theirs for the world. So, could I help fix up this manuscript so that others could read it and benefit from their experience?

It was a pleasure.

Fred Hill
Charlestown, Indiana

FORWARD

Like most couples in their early forties, our life settled into a somewhat comfortable routine. We were no different than most couples with children who are involved with different school activities and ball games to attend. Our lives focused on our children and these activities. Making sure we attended their games and programs at school, chauffeuring them to and from appointments and commitments: these are the happy details from which a contented life emerges. Although it's all a chore at times, we really wouldn't have it any other way.

Then one day, after a routine yearly mammogram, our whole world changed. What used to be the most important things in our life now took a back seat to real life worries and concerns.

This is my story about my breast cancer told through my husband's eyes. He started out writing his thoughts and feelings down as therapy for himself. But, as doctors visits mounted and concerns grew he decided to tell our story in hopes that it might shed new light on a couple's problem. That's right. When a loved one is stricken with some disease or affliction, it does become a couple's problem.

Too many times the spouses are asked to sit on the sidelines and give good moral support to their spouse. This is where our story differs from most people. We have always been there for one another through good times and bad. This is why our wedding vows say, "for richer or poorer, in sickness and in health, till death do us part." That's our belief. Being involved with each other has been very important in our marriage.

My husband wrote this book not only as therapy for himself, but with the hope that more husbands will become involved with the care of their wife. In his profession as a funeral director, he has seen so many instances where there is so little conversation between spouses about an illness.

Our story does not end in death. It ends in hope and with a future together. Our story ends this way only because we both believe in early detection. Even though this was the most difficult time to go through in our life, our life together is better because of it. That may be hard for some readers to understand, but it is true. Our cancer trials and tribulations have in fact refocused our attention into those things that are truly important.

Karen Grayson
Charlestown, Indiana
February 13, 2002

B	ack in 1975 I was a pretty good high school basketball player in New Washington, Indiana. We lived in a small farming community about 25 miles northeast of Louisville, Kentucky. Living in this small town, yet near to a large city, we shared the advantages of both. But we preferred the somewhat slower paced community of New Washington, where you knew everyone. People left their doors unlocked at night and felt safe doing so. The attractions of the big city were only a 30-minute drive away, but when you headed for home, you left all the city's problems behind you.

New Washington High School awarded diplomas to only 42 students at the end of my senior year. The intimate setting of this small school and peaceful community allowed us to form close, long-term relationships with classmates. We shared good times and bad times, and even shared those personal matters we might have preferred to keep to ourselves. There was comfort and a sense of security among us, but we knew that we would soon have to select our separate paths of life. I had to choose a college where I would continue my basketball and educational career.

Long-term plans suddenly demanded our attention around graduation time. I planned to continue my education for only one more year, before returning home to enter mortuary school. My dream had always been to join the family business after college. My family has owned a funeral business since 1949 and my life's ambition was to be a funeral director. I'm sure my father and grandfather planned to pass the business to an offspring one day, and as the oldest grandchild I was the logical choice. I had always enjoyed spending weekends with my grandparents. I especially enjoyed learning the family business and gaining responsibilities in it, just as a young kid might start off as a stock boy in his dad's department store. I enjoyed the opportunity to work with my grandfather on funerals and going with him on ambulance runs.

Until the late 70s, most funeral homes provided ambulance service to their communities and surrounding areas. In small towns like Charlestown and New Washington, this was more of a civic duty than a profit venture. Expensive equipment was beyond our reach, as was expensively trained personnel. Instead, we provided quick response to an emergency and concentrated on the application of bandages, splints and oxygen. The drama of each emergency, the importance of our work and the need for speed made ambulance runs an exciting adventure for a boy my age, and my grandfather believed that this was a valuable experience for me.

My parents were uncomfortable with some of this. A day at work with Grandpa exposed me to sights and situations they felt I wasn't ready to see. My grandpa felt otherwise; he used a special signal to notify me he was about to leave on an ambulance run. He would wink and nod his head a certain way and I knew that meant we had a run. I would then go hide on the floorboard of the ambulance until we were off the parking lot and out of sight. He would then tell me the coast was clear. Only then would I sit up straight and enjoy the excitement and drama of emergency work.

I grew up quickly on Grandpa's ambulance runs. As an impressionable kid, I learned about a lot of things ahead of my time. A small town emergency worker sees plenty of terror and tragedy, often involving friends, neighbors and relatives. We were called to auto accidents, suicides, heart attacks, fires, and every form of death from sudden collapse to the final breath of a long-suffering disease victim. I remember being particularly sorry for the cancer victims I saw, because the slow torture of pain seemed intolerable and unfair to me. Of all the pain I saw, cancer left the strongest impression.

Not all of this drama involved death, of course. I was awakened one night and rushed off to a sudden childbirth. Too young to know the details surrounding these events, I only remember the shocking images

I saw: a streetlight shining on the sidewalk, well after midnight; the distended stomach of the frightened woman; her screams that the baby was coming out. I caught the urge to scream from her, and demanded that Grandpa get her to the hospital fast. As I said, I grew up quick on those runs.

I also learned the frustrations of emergency personnel. We lacked the equipment sometimes needed and couldn't offer the services of a trained paramedic. I can remember riding with patients who screamed in agony and pleaded for something to stop their pain, while we could do little more than rush them to the emergency room. These moments of medical impotency also effected me strongly—the empty feeling of sitting helplessly beside of a person whose suffering you can do nothing to stop.

Throughout high school, I worked along with my brother Jeff in the family business. Although we were the owners' children and grandchildren, we still had to start at the bottom. Entry-level candidates had to cut the grass at the funeral homes and the cemetery. Whenever my father offered our services, we also mowed the yards of family or friends. Dad rarely told anybody no—he genuinely enjoyed helping others, and believed it was also good for business. Jeff and I didn't always see it that way. We also dug graves and shoveled snow when necessary. In other words, we learned the business from the bottom up.

The demands of the funeral business kept us too busy to enjoy a normal adolescent life. The death care industry is a 24-hour operation: we were expected to attend school daily and work daily. Only when both duties were done could we interact with our friends. We were always allowed to participate in any sports activities we wanted. But whenever we weren't at school, we had work to do.

This responsibility to our family business didn't provide me with much of an opportunity to study the opposite sex. I was just shy enough to accept this arrangement for the time being. But I do remember asking the good Lord to provide me with an opportunity to meet a young lady while in college and begin developing a relationship with her. I even went so far as to specify the type of girl I wanted to date and eventually marry. Like any young healthy basketball player, I naturally wanted a blond-haired, beautiful cheerleader to have an interest in me. If I could get this one wish while in college, I thought my future would be set. Sadly, every other healthy young male in Indiana chose the same criteria, and the waiting list must have been quite long. My request went unanswered for quite some time.

Along with the end of my high school studies came the end of my high school basketball career. Here, too, I had to make some decisions about the future. My coach, Mike Sandifar, met with my family and me one Sunday afternoon to discuss the various schools that had recruited me. Scouts and coaches had showed some interest in my services, and we now plowed through a pile of recruiting brochures, letters, and propaganda. We narrowed down the list of schools by eliminating all the big schools and the junior colleges. I eventually settled on taking a trip to Kansas to look at a couple of colleges out there.

The trip was long and tiring and Kansas looked very flat and foreign. It seemed too far away from home and family. After visiting a few schools I still didn't know where to further my education and basketball careers.

We started towards home after a couple of days, driving through Missouri and southern Illinois. Endless, redundant prairie rolled by my window, and I sank into silence. My coach and I had run out of things to talk about on this long trip, and I became absorbed in worried thoughts about the future. During one of these quiet times I began to have thoughts about a college in McKenzie, TN called Bethel College. It was almost as if someone was speaking to me. It was not a voice I could hear but more of a feeling that I had in my head and heart.

A former New Washington High School player and great friend of mine, Lynn Sanders, had already enrolled at Bethel and was on their basketball team. Yet I hadn't really considered going to school there. I had never seen the school and had only talked to the assistant coaches once when they came to see me play one night. They didn't seem too impressed with me at the time. I'd left town after the game to go get a pizza with some of my friends. We had just ordered our meal when I received a call from my mother telling me there was a coach to see me. She suggested that I come home immediately. I was upset. I did what I was told, but I'm sure the coaches felt my resentment. I didn't give him the time of day. The school never followed up with an offer, and I gave them no further thought.

Now, driving through barren southern Illinois months later, this unexplained voice in my head demanded my attention. 'Go visit Bethel,' it insisted for what seemed like hours. Not really understanding any of this, I told coach Sandifar that I wanted to visit Bethel College.

Coach Sandifar knew how fickle a frightened teenager could be when facing the future. He said, "You realize this college is not on your original list of schools to visit. But it does meet your requirements, if you want to take a look at it."

I knew I wasn't making much sense, but I told him, "I really think I would like to at least see the place before eliminating it altogether." He patiently indulged me and helped schedule a visit.

Soon we hit the road again, window-shopping for my future. I was naturally nervous about leaving home and trying to fit in somewhere else. Could I find new friends in another state, succeed in my classes and contribute to a college basketball team? Lots of uncertainty lurked before me.

The campus visit quickly reassured me. Bethel Coach Lionel Sinn took us on a tour. It was exactly what I had hoped for. The school had a small enrollment and the setting seemed intimate; no enormous lecture halls where a freshman from a farm town might get lost.

When we completed our tour, we stood outside the library while Coach Sinn wrapped up his tour. His concluding remarks were not designed to close the deal. "I can not guarantee you the school will be open in the fall." He went on to explain the school had had some financial trouble and was really on shaky ground. They had recruited

Bob Hope for a Memorial Day fund-raiser, which he agreed to do as a favor to one of the trustees of the school. The coach had been honest enough to share these concerns before I made a final decision, but he also seemed confident that Bethel would hold on. I concluded my visit by playing a pick-up game with some of the current team members. It was just what I wanted—a chance to work off some steam and see how I shaped up against some prospective teammates.

As soon as I stepped onto the court for this pick-up game, I heard this voice inside me once again. It told me this was the place for me and I was good enough for this team. For the next hour that we played, something just came over me. I surprised myself and swept aside all uncertainty. My game seemed to step up to the next level automatically. My moves and shots flowed easily and effectively, although I knew I was playing beyond my ability. This was most exhilarating.

I walked off the court, thinking that this was the place for me. The silent voice inside me nagged me until I closed the deal. Just a week after returning home from my visit to Bethel, I followed this voice and decided to attend Bethel College in McKenzie, Tennessee.

The first step away from a somewhat sheltered life can be scary for a high school senior from small-town Indiana. But as summer began to fade, about the time school began, this persistent voice returned and reassured me that things were going to be just fine. We drove down to McKenzie, unpacked my bags and settled into college life. As classes began and basketball practice started up, I found a comfortable routine. I adjusted well and began to make a few friends on the team and around campus.

The college game demands practice seven days a week—one of those adjustments I had to make. More commitment and less recovery time or leisure; totally different from the part-time demands of high school basketball. Studying and keeping up with course work absorbed the rest of my time, leaving little opportunity for socializing.

The first real break from basketball came at Christmas. As a naïve college freshman, I looked forward to at least a week off. After our last game before Christmas on the 22nd of December, Coach Sinn walked in and recommended that we, "enjoy the Christmas break and be ready and on the court for practice starting December 26, at 6 PM." The dreaded two-a-days (double workout sessions) would begin on the next day and continue through New Years Day. He was planning to hold practice sessions at 10 AM and at 6 PM. These were the hard facts of life at the next level.

Before we left for our Christmas mini-break, all the players had to pack up everything we needed—clothes, sheets, shaving cream and so on—and move into some other dorm. In those days, all the dorms were closed for cleaning except one. Everyone staying on campus during the break had to move into one dorm.

I returned from the Christmas break and settled into my new room and got ready for practice. My roommate for this week was my best friend Lynn Sanders. Lynn was a sophomore and knew his way around campus and the town of McKenzie more that I. He was also more outgoing than I was at this point in my life.

McKenzie is a small town of about 7,000 people; a quiet community in western Tennessee. Like New Washington, there aren't many entertainment options in the evenings. And it's just as well, since we received a mere $10 a day for meals. After our second practice of the day, the tired ballplayers trudged back to the dorm for the glamorous leisure of college basketball stars: watching a black-and-white portable TV that only received one station. The rest of the campus was empty and quiet. Our classmates were sleeping late at home, catching up on their meals and laundry, congratulating themselves for not trying out for the basketball team.

After our first practice session on the 26th of December, we were all winded and reminded that we needed work before the season resumed. Christmas break loomed ahead of me like a dreary boot camp. So I was open for suggestions when Lynn shared some inside information.

"There's a girl that would like to go out with you." I guess he knew I would never discover this fact for myself. "Her name is Karen Beal and she's a blonde cheerleader for the team."

My mood changed immediately. I recalled that shopping list I had given the Lord, and wondered if this was the love interest that had been on back order for some time. Lynn knew I needed a game plan and a little coaching. "Chris, you know this girl. Since there is so little to do in the evenings, I want to know if you will at least talk to her."

How could I tell him I would prefer joining a bunch of sweaty off-duty athletes huddling around a TV set in the rec room? But in fact, I didn't know this girl at all. Newly arrived freshman keep much too busy and way too intimidated to form any designs on the cheerleading squad.

Here was an invitation to climb out of my shell. With only a little hesitation, I agreed to go out with her.

All day on the 27th I tried to pump Lynn for more information about Karen. After all, a worldly upperclassman and a known fixture on the basketball squad should have all the pertinent facts regarding the cheerleaders. Lynn could only provide the basics: she lived in McKenzie. Further intelligence was hard to find. Contact between male and female students was no easy matter in those days. Bethel College is sponsored by the Cumberland Presbyterian Church and they did their best to contain the fires of pre-marital curiosity. Back in 1975 a coed had to be signed out to leave the dorm for the evening and had to return at a specified time. Girls were not permitted to visit the men's dorm at any time. Karen and a friend were scheduled to meet us at 7 PM.

Finally, at 7 PM on December 27, 1975 I met Karen Beal. When she knocked on the window of our room I immediately felt very nervous. Where was that interior voice that had been so eager to instruct me during other times of stress? I raised the window shade to answer the knock, already bending the tight moral codes of the college. I then accepted delivery on the package I had ordered. All my specifications checked out: a cheerleader, blond hair, very beautiful. Every other Midwestern male my age could eat his heart out.

I fell in love with Karen very quickly. Those plans to return to Indiana next year and enroll in mortuary college now lay crumpled up on the floor. I had shed the skin of a frightened freshman: now I was a sophisticated college student, a starter on the basketball team, relishing the further distinction of dating a cheerleader. In short, I was actually enjoying my time away from home and the family business. That voice that led me to Bethel had not steered me wrong: my prayers had been answered.

That lonely, abandoned campus now seemed like a much happier place to me. Over the next several days Karen and I began spending more and more time together. She showed me around town and introduced me to her parents. We found our own entertainment, apart from the student social activities. By now the rest of the student body had returned from Christmas break, but Karen and I spent our precious leisure time off-campus. The guys in the dorm would just have to watch that black-and-white TV without me.

Somehow through all this happy distraction I managed to go to class, pass my tests, hand in most of my papers and show some progress on the basketball court. I also went home on weekends when I could, and kept up with the family business. I guess Dad decided I was now ready for the facts of life, because I joined him now for occasional ambulance runs.

One Saturday while I was home, we received a call concerning a man who was apparently suffering a heart attack at a local gas station. My father and I rushed off in the ambulance, and I discovered that the patient was the father of one of my classmates. He walked out of the station by himself and climbed onto our cot and we took off on the 25-mile trip to the nearest emergency room.

As we hurried toward the hospital, this man's condition deteriorated rapidly. All we could offer him was some oxygen and the quickest trip possible. I sat at my usual post beside the patient, watching him fight for the breath he needed while his face faded to a purplish color. He begged me to help him breathe, gasping and gesturing his desperation to me, kicking his legs and surrendering to panic. There was nothing I could do. He died five miles from the hospital, right next to me. I remember watching the ER doctors and nurses hopelessly trying to bring him back. And I sank into a depression of guilt and helplessness, remaining within that cloud for several days

But life and love soon called me back. Once the weather warmed up, Karen and I purchased 10-speed bikes and spent a lot of time riding our bikes with Karen's brother Charles and his wife Kay. We rode all over the city of McKenzie and sometimes way out into the country. My priorities were changing, and this became apparent even in my waistline. Previously my day had revolved around suppertime, but now I was too much in love to waste time eating. From the end of the basketball season in February to the end of the semester in May, my weight dropped from 232 pounds to 198. I was hardly ever spotted in the school cafeteria that spring and spent most of my time after school at Charles and Kay's home. My friends could see quite a change in me.

Anyone who saw us together knew what was coming next. Dreading a long summer of separation after several months of dating, we set the date to get married on June 11, 1977. We informed our families and asked for their blessing. Along with this approval, my grandmother shared some advice: "Remember that marriage is forever. There will be some disagreements and difficult times for you throughout your life. But if you can always be there for each other, your marriage will be very successful."

Karen and I smiled back at my grandmother. She had earned the right to preach about marriage after enjoying her own fine marriage, and I had never known her to be shy about sharing her wisdom. She then surprised us by requesting one thing. "If you are planning on June 11th for a wedding, you can surely wait one more day and get married on Sunday June 12."

Did she think these impulsive kids couldn't wait an extra day? Was this some sort of cooling-off period to test our commitment to each other? I had to ask, "Why do you want us to wait one more day?"

"Because June 12th is your grandparents' wedding anniversary and we would like for you to get married the same day." Fortunately we hadn't selected a weekend in October. It was my grandmother's way of giving us her blessing. We both quickly agreed.

As I have said, my priorities were quickly changing, and the plans I had made for my life no longer applied. Karen convinced me to stay in school and get my teaching degree. The more I was away from the funeral business, the more I liked my free time. I decided it would be nice to teach and coach a little basketball for about 5 years before going back home to the family business. I changed my major to Health, Physical Education and Recreation, and both of us decided to minor in sociology. Our intentions here were not necessarily academic: sharing a minor meant spending more time with each other. We had several classes together and we had a professor who was a big basketball fan. He taught 8 AM classes and took pity on the tough schedule of a college athlete. If we had a late game he would tell me to sleep in and have Karen come to class and get the notes. It worked out just fine—she took better notes than me anyway.

Karen finished her elementary education degree in 1978 and got a teaching job in Huntington, Tennessee. This meant we had to move there. She taught one year while I commuted to school and finished my degree. One semester of student teaching helped me to decide that teaching was not for me.

Instead, I had changed my mind about becoming a funeral director. All that time spent working with my grandfather had left an impression on me, and I decided that the family business was right for me. Karen was not particularly happy with my decision, especially after she learned that I turned down an offer to be a graduate assistant at a university in Missouri. One of Karen's dreams was to be the wife of a coach. She really likes sports and would have made a great coach's wife.

Few young men from Indiana could resist a wife with such ambitions. But I didn't want to teach, and she could tell where my heart was.

So it was back to Indiana, enroll in mortuary school and re-join the family business, adjust to a new marriage and start a family on a shoestring budget. College students often get shaken up on the rough landing from the heights of academic life to the realities of the working world. We hit a few bumps too and had to work hard just to get through each day as it came. We would barely clear one obstacle before turning to face an even bigger one ahead. In 1980, our first son Michael was born; six years later Michelle came along, followed by Stephen in 1989. Things weren't always easy for us, but we were well on our way toward "living happily ever after."

It was a warm day in June 2000 when we encountered our biggest, most unexpected obstacle on the road to happiness. Karen went for her annual mammogram at the Women's Diagnostic Center in Louisville. This was a routine visit: a good habit of personal maintenance. She felt comfortable going to this particular clinic because they specialize in this important and often uncomfortable procedure. There are doctors on staff who will give you the results of your mammogram before you leave. Other places make you wait a week or two wondering about the results, but at the Women's Diagnostic Center, a healthy woman like Karen can submit to the inconvenience and discomfort, receive her passing grade and then move on to the more pressing business of her life.

Karen arrived home late that afternoon. She began sorting through the mail, weeding out the junk and examining the bills. I came home about an hour later, tired from a day at the office and ready to relax. I gave the mail a quick glance as usual, decided the lawn could afford to grow another inch or so and went back to our bedroom to change my clothes. My immediate schedule called for something cold to drink on the patio around our pool and some therapeutic relaxation before fixing supper.

Karen came out by the pool and we starting talking about each other's day. She waited for me to ask about her check-up, but I didn't think to do so. "Since you didn't ask about my appointment, I will tell you anyway." She described the routine of the late afternoon appointment, registering at the desk, and then waiting to see the doctor. "When the doctor came in, he examined me and we then looked at the films together."

The Doctor stared into the light silhouetting the image of the examined tissue, with an eye trained to look for details the rest of us cannot interpret. His silent gaze at the film was intense and worrisome. "There is a area of concern and something looks different from last year's films," Dr. McLaughlin finally said with a slight frown. "I'd like for you to go back across the hall for another mammogram and I will tell the technician to focus on the particular area in question."

Karen showed no alarm about the need for a follow-up examination. Years ago she had needed a second x-ray because of mastitis. It seemed reasonable to assume that this follow-up measure was a precautionary measure.

But after examining the second mammogram, the doctor felt sure that something was wrong. Karen had gone there alone, and afterwards described what transpired while I sat on the edge of my seat. He had reported some suspicion to Karen; a change in the readings, an area of some concern. Dr. McLaughlin recommended an ultrasound to provide a better comparison between this mammogram and the one taken in March of 1999. "Some of the tissues look suspicious," he said simply, in a quiet voice that nonetheless thundered inside Karen's head.

Dr. McLaughlin went on to say, "A biopsy will have to be done to determine the exact makeup of this suspicious area." His tone of voice smothered any sense of panic under a comforting cover, as if he were conducting routine business. But he knew the emotional impact of words like "lesion" and "biopsy". "Do you have a surgeon you prefer to do the biopsy, or would you like me to make an appointment with one I recommend?"

As he compared the two x-rays in minute detail, it seemed to her that his voice faded into an echo. Her concentration strangely wandered. While the doctor rattled off the medical details to Karen, some sort of numbing fog rose around her, some sort of surpassing reality that took precedence over the moment. I wouldn't learn until later that my wife already believed she had breast cancer.

Karen felt herself sinking under the weight of his words. She heard "surgeon" and "biopsy" and heard those terrifying terms reverberate inside her. The doctor had to repeat his question before Karen replied that she hadn't had need of one before now. She had to rally to offer a response: "I'll go to anyone you recommend." Dr. McLaughlin called the team at Surgical Associates of Louisville.

The doctor he requested was unavailable for a month or so. Dr. McLaughlin didn't want to wait that long. Instead, an appointment was scheduled with Dr. Richard Pokorny.

Karen drove herself to the mammogram appointment, and returned home with plenty on her mind. She usually worries about fighting rush hour traffic, but on this day the traffic must have disappeared, because she made it back to Charlestown in record time. Should she call me on the phone to tell me how the visit went? No, this was too important and needed to be shared face to face. Over and over she rehearsed in her mind how to announce the news of the latest procedure. Facing a gathering crisis in her own health, her mind focused only on how to reassure her husband.

As Karen relayed this ominous news to me, she tried to adopt the doctor's tone of voice, so businesslike and emotionless. Her clinical description betrayed no particular fear. But the first tremors of terror were close to the surface. I tried to show concern without allowing any alarm to slip out, but I doubt that I succeeded in this. Karen went on to tell me the doctor had scheduled the ultrasound for Thursday June 29, 2000. Since he needed more precise diagnostic details, the doctor wouldn't venture to speculate what all this meant. These were scattered fibro-glandular densities that could obscure a lesion.

I felt a banging inside my heart, as if someone had just slammed the screen door and broken into our house. That "happily-ever-after" ending had suddenly been thrown into doubt by complications too scary to consider. The mind so quickly leaps into negativity and imagines the worst. With such frightening possibilities now on the table, it seemed impossible to wait for yet another test. How long will it be before we know anything for certain?

Karen grew skilled at briefing me in a calm, detached manner. Clearly she was concerned over how worried I had become. "Dr. McLaughlin tried to get me in for the ultrasound today. He said I need it to accurately determine the size of the area in question. The technician was gone for the day. So I have it scheduled for the 29th." It sounded as routine as an appointment at the beauty salon.

Karen was handling the stress better than I was, at least at this point. I was devastated, to an extent that alarmed her. She just wanted to get all this diagnostic work over with, get her suspicions confirmed, and move on toward treatment. I, on the other hand, felt like a bystander watching an accident approaching, feeling unable to prevent it. Clouds were gathering for a looming storm, and I could only watch and worry.

On Thursday June 29, Karen went for her ultrasound appointment at Women's Diagnostics Center in Louisville, KY. After the procedure, the technician told Karen, "I knew the doctors were good but I didn't know they were this good! This was the smallest lump I have ever seen detected. If I had not been given the general location to look for it, it might not have been detected with the ultrasound." Whether or not this statement was actually true, it was a comfort to Karen to know it had been detected at the earliest stage possible.

After waiting a short period of time, Dr. McLaughlin called Karen into a room where he had the mammogram results and the ultrasound findings. Dr. McLaughlin then said, "Upon closer examination of the area in question, I find a mass measuring 12 millimeters with speculated margins in the anterior upper region of the right breast, along with an oval mass measuring 6 millimeters with circumscribed margins seen in the middle lateral region of the same breast." These figures meant nothing to Karen at first. He then began to explain the importance of finding the mass at such a small size and began talking about survivor rates with such an early detection if the biopsy were to indicate the mass was in fact malignant.

I asked all the questions I could think of about how the ultrasound went and provided all the assurance I could muster. We predictably agreed that the biopsy was necessary and might clear up the whole thing. Even platitudes like "better safe than sorry" crept into our conversations, but these didn't seem too convincing. Both of us tried to remain positive—everything we had learned was strictly preliminary—but we didn't indulge in denial. This was no time for panic. Plenty of concern, perhaps, but no panic.

We tried to carry on our home life without raising our children's concerns. There seemed to be no need to worry them until something was certain. All these doctor visits were explained as routine mainte-nance and attended to along with the other mundane errands of family life. But our daughter Michelle sensed something in all this. She is very sensitive to anything out of the ordinary or out of place, and couldn't be fooled by our charade.

"I have another appointment scheduled for July," Karen told her, offering the truth if not the whole truth.

"You just got back from the doctor," she protested. "Why all of these appointments all of a sudden?"

"It just seems that way. It's summer break. I have to schedule all my doctor visits when school is not in session, that's all."

She smelled a rat. "No one has this many doctor's appointments unless something is wrong." Her eyes demanded an answer. "Mom, what's wrong with you?"

The truth came out. But they agreed to keep it from the boys until something was known for sure.

The next phase started a week later. I was unable to go with Karen for her first consultation with Dr. Pokorny, so she asked our friend Becky Zimmerman to accompany her. Dr. Pokorny outlined the cur-rent plan of action to determine just what this mass was. "I suggest a stereotactic biopsy of the upper-outer quadrant of the right breast at Baptist East Hospital in Louisville on July 10." He then explained this procedure in graphic detail: "A stereotactic biopsy consists of a small needle inserted into the mass with the help of a computer. The sample will be removed and sent to pathology for examination. You will need to report to the hospital at about 2 PM. and the procedure will be done at 3 PM. It lasts approximately 45 minutes. A 1% solution of Lidocaine will be given to anesthetize the area and a small incision will be made to allow the needle to penetrate the skin and then the mass.

You will be lying face down on a table with your breast hanging through a hole in the table so the computer can attach itself and perform the biopsy."

Karen received these details more bravely than I. I believe that it is best to have all the information you can get, to understand the situation and your options while avoiding the fear of the unknown. There is even something reassuring in the chance to immerse yourself in details, rather than squander your thoughts on the terrifying implications. But this frank description was hard to take. The closest a man can come to understanding what all this feels like would be to picture being the patient in an analogous situation. Imagine your most intimate, vulnerable appendage(s) hanging through a hole on an operating table, attached to a computer while a needle penetrates deeply to remove a threatening mass of tissue. I found no reassurance in such thoughts.

This was my first time to get really worried. Now we were suddenly facing the possibility of cancer. Hearing Karen report the doctor's words made me realize that it would have been more reassuring for me if I could have accompanied her to the doctor's office. The demands of work had left me no choice, but I didn't like the helpless feeling of being a spectator while matters became more and more serious. Karen didn't seem to be particularly worried at this point, but I think I was worried enough for both of us. I vowed to myself to let nothing interfere with my active involvement.

We went to the hospital together on July 10th. A registration associate walked us through the necessary paperwork and took a copy of our insurance card. She then directed us to the area where the stereotactic biopsy would be performed. We registered there and took our seats amidst a waiting room full of worried people.

After several minutes, a nurse announced to us that the doctor was tied up in surgery and would be about an hour late. She reviewed for us once again how the procedure would be performed and asked if we had any questions.

I spoke up. "Will I be able to watch this biopsy take place?"

"Watch?" The nurse laughed at my naïve request. "It is not permitted." This appeared to be the standard answer, given to me without consideration or discussion. My concern was touching, perhaps, but not appropriate. Her hand gesture suggested that I should sit back down and stay out of the way while they resume their important work.

So I sat back down, confused and frustrated. My wife would face the most frightening episode of her life all alone, while I sat on the sidelines and waited for the outcome. So much for my determination to get more involved in all this, I thought. I shuffled my feet impatiently and probably muttered to myself. It was my first taste of the indifference of medical personnel and facilities to the patient's family.

I tried to remind myself of the doctor's point of view, in my more generous moments. Their primary concern is the health and recovery of the patient; I didn't question that. But how about some consideration and support for the spouse and family? I needed to participate in order to contribute something to Karen's support and care. I felt completely separated from the whole procedure.

Instead, I faced a room full of silent relatives, all deeply concerned with what was happening to their loved ones behind those closed doors. We were all rendered irrelevant, shunted aside and sedated with the standard waiting room diversions: a soap opera on the TV, shopworn issues of *People* magazine, redundant coded messages on the intercom. My frustration quickly kindled into anger.

When someone you love is undergoing tests that might show cancer, anyone's nerves would be on edge. It doesn't matter if the doctor believes the results will be negative or not—you still have this nervous feeling until you find out the answer. The patient is permitted an active role in this process and a chance to ask questions, offer input, and express concerns. Their fears will be acknowledged and addressed; their rights and feelings will be respected. As painful as the patient's position can be, he or she is at least allowed the involvement that lends some feeling of control over the situation.

Karen recognized this disparity when we spoke about it later. The spouse is the one on the bench. While the life of a loved one might be on the line behind a flimsy curtain, we are expected to distract ourselves with an old magazine. One of the nurses summed up my situation bluntly: "About all you can do is to be a chauffeur for her at this time."

We decided to walk outside so Karen could grab one last smoke before the biopsy. When we returned, we sat in the waiting room for about a half-hour until the nurse called her back. During the entire time the procedure was taking place, I sat feebly in the waiting room and skimmed my way through gossip sheets and photos of the evening gowns at the Academy Awards. I think I was grinding my teeth. It is a terrible feeling to want to participate in the care of your loved one and then not be allowed.

The biopsy took approximately 45 minutes. Immediately after it was over, the doctor came out to speak to me. This was my first meeting with Dr. Pokorny: he appeared to be young and very professional. He gave me a very cautious assessment of the situation. "I can tell nothing from this procedure at this time. There is no point in speculating. All answers will have to wait until the lab work is done." We would have to wait until we meet on the 12th to hear about the lab results. Only then could he interpret the data, explain our options and suggest what should come next. "Karen will be out in just a few minutes. She will need to keep her arm bent and across her chest for the next 24 hours. An ice bag on the area will relieve any possible swelling or bruising over the next 24 hours. She must avoid lifting anything with that arm for several days. She has been instructed to leave the bandage on until it comes off by itself, which should be in about a week."

Karen came out shakily and we went directly home. On the way home, she tried to explain to me how the procedure was performed. We talked back and forth about what our options might be for the future. We both felt a powerful impatience to know the results immediately and the frustration of not being able to find out.

Over the next 24 hours Karen was a really good patient. She followed the doctor's orders exactly and did not appear to be in a tremendous amount of pain. She was willing to talk to our friends that stopped by or called on the phone.

The next several days were emotionally difficult for both of us. Now that my wife had had a surgical procedure performed on her breast, my mind started working overtime. I became consumed with the worst case scenario. Since I'm a funeral director, this attitude is only natural. I see only the worst cases, and see them in rather graphic detail. With this perspective, I could imagine only one outcome. Of course, I had heard about the good cases where surgery has removed the cancer and drugs and therapy had halted or reversed the advance. But my personal experience has been with the terminal cases, and this tended to influence my attitude.

I started placing myself in the position of some of the families I was currently serving. Would my face soon show the same grief, the same wrenching sense of loss I see so often in my line of work? Who will help me through all this? Who comforts the comforter when he endures the loss of a loved one? It became increasingly difficult for me to disassociate myself from my worst thoughts.

It took an effort to shake off these dark premonitions, which I realized were generated by a sense of self-pity. They did nothing to help Karen. But even when the most morbid thoughts subsided, there was plenty to worry about. Breast cancer strikes at an especially intimate target, a portion of a woman's anatomy that represents nourishing and nurturing of offspring, as well as her own attractiveness and sexuality. I also began wondering how Karen would react to the small scar on her breast. Would she feel different about herself and would that affect our relationship sexually? I told myself that I wasn't in love with her breast, but with her. Was I being honest with myself? And how would Karen see all this?

During this time we were left with all these thoughts while waiting on the results of the biopsy. In the beginning, I thought I was handling the situation okay. But the strains of waiting and uncertainty became progressively greater. I remember Bill Cosby explaining how his father administered punishment: "Next Thursday, you're gonna get a whipping." The anticipation multiplied the pain, until it weighed him down like an impending death sentence. I felt a similar, accumulating sense of dread.

Finally, the day arrived when we would see the results. All day leading up to that moment, I deliberately tried to keep a positive attitude. It seemed to be the longest day ever, made longer by a mind that refused to focus on anything but the impending appointment. We met with Dr. Pokorny at 2 PM on Wednesday July 12.

This date was already significant to me, because this was the ten-year anniversary of my grandfather's death. He died July 12, 1990 at age 80 as a result of complications from lung cancer. This is just the sort of coincidence that leads the mind to gloomy associations and unhealthy conclusions. I was with my grandfather the night the doctor told him he thought he might have cancer. I can remember the doctor telling him they wanted to do a biopsy on his lung to confirm his suspicions. When the doctor very bluntly told my grandfather how they would perform this biopsy and then follow up with chemotherapy and radiation, I remember Grandpa telling the doctor he was not going to have anything done. He preferred to take his chances. "I've seen the results of chemotherapy and radiation on people and how they had been burnt," he declared, citing that mortician's perspective. "I'm not willing to go through all that."

I had always been very close to my grandfather, and had already mourned this anniversary for ten years. Now a new gloom was joining the old one. Would we be in this same situation by the end of the day? Would fearful scenarios and agonizing options occupy our thoughts from now on? Would we have to make similar tough decisions at the young age of 43?

We arrived at Dr. Pokorny's office, registered and waited about 10 minutes. Then a nurse called us into the examination room. She instructed my wife to disrobe above the waist and put on this hospital gown. "Dr. Pokorny will be examining the breast to see how the scar from the stereotactic biopsy is healing."

Karen sat and waited in silence, either consumed by her thoughts or firmly resisting them. We were both in a non-talkative mood. We had already talked this subject to death and there was nothing to do but wait. Dr. Pokorny was running a few minutes late and he apologized to us as he came into the room. We quickly exchanged pleasantries and he got right to the point. "The pathological result came back inconclusive. I cannot rule out the possibility that this spot is cancer. There are indications that some tissues are tubular in nature. This could be consistent with cancer, but it is not always the case."

Is lingering uncertainty the worst outcome of all? I stole a glance at my wife. Karen's face betrayed emotions I had never seen before. She looked hollow, drained, her hopes sank inside her. The courage that had propped her up during this long wait now seemed to collapse momentarily. Our emotions started to run rampant because now the possibility of having breast cancer just increased. A thousand questions assaulted my mind, along with a list of unthinkable consequences from mastectomy to chemotherapy to death.

The doctor outlined the next step we faced: "You will need another surgical procedure called a needle localization biopsy. This procedure will also have to be performed as an outpatient at the hospital, and it involves the operating room and sedation." He described the procedure with precision, knowing that such frankness is more bearable than uncertainty. "There will be an incision of about 2 to 2 1/2 inches. It will take about 45 minutes to complete. A needle will be inserted into the area of the mass and then a more thorough biopsy can be completed. The samples will be sent to pathology and we will know the results within a few days." Once again he chose his words carefully, unable to answer the question foremost in our minds: "Like before, I cannot tell without lab work whether or not this is a definite cancer.

But in 80% of the cases that are similar to Karen's, the results come back negative for cancer."

This final estimate appeared to be our ray of hope and best possible news of the day. Even so, our odds had dropped to one in five.

We spent the next hour and fifteen minutes with Doctor Pokorny, who endured our questions and concerns without allowing any interruption. We went over the entire range of possibilities, from not having cancer to the possible treatments in the event it was cancer. We speculated about possible causes. My wife is a smoker, smoking about a pack a day. Our kids and I have encouraged her to quit for several years without success. So my first question focused on this possible connection. "Could this possible cancer be caused from Karen's smoking?"

"The chance of that being the case is minimal. I am more concerned with her having heart disease, a stroke or lung cancer from smoking, but not breast cancer". He didn't miss the opportunity to tell her how important it is for her to quit. No one wants to know that his or her health crisis was self-induced and avoidable. Knowing that smoking probably didn't cause the situation we were in somehow made me feel better. I had always feared that, at some point in our lives if she didn't stop smoking, we would eventually get to the point where cancer would invade our lives. It would have been hard to face the guilt that might come from the realization that if we had been more strident in expressing our concerns, this problem might never have appeared. But this relief hardly countered our more serious concerns just now.

Dr. Pokorny described all the possible treatments that might be applied if this biopsy was identified as cancerous. Options ranged from doing nothing to chemotherapy and radiation, mastectomy and breast reconstruction. The truth hurt, of course, but it left us with a full understanding of the options and consequences available to us. It also empowered us to take an active, intelligent role in the decisions that would have to be made.

I soon realized just how important knowledge is for the patient and family members. Ignorance and uncertainty can only lead to panic and poor choices. The patient and her family must educate themselves if they want to be able to ask intelligent questions and to follow-up with the doctor.

No doctor can guess your thoughts and concerns or judge your confusion and misconceptions. The patient and supporting family members must press the issue by trying to get into a dialogue with the doctor. Too many of us are intimidated in a doctor's office. We are silenced by the fear of asking a dumb question or taking up too much of a professional's important time. The haste of some physicians to move on to the next patient can also discourage a timid patient, making them leave the office without a clear idea of the problems they might face.

This intimidation factor also causes many patients to accept a doctor's assessment without challenge or analysis. Most doctors are not going to go into any more detail than they have to; few will offer countering arguments or dissenting research. Instead, it is too easy to hide behind a mantle of authority and offer a few observations without differentiating between fact and opinion. Like the timid car owner at a mechanic's mercy, too many patients just accept what the doctor is saying as gospel. They do not ask follow up questions or ask why the doctor has decided on one particular path of treatment over another. And without securing such assurance, the patient might remain unconvinced; undermining the cooperation needed to carry out their end of the treatment. We have a tendency to forget that a doctor is just *practicing* medicine.

Medical treatment is not yet an exact science. The doctor with the best intentions still doesn't have all the answers. All parties involved in caring for and supporting a person in a medical concern have a profound responsibility to educate themselves, prepare for these appointments ahead of time and not be afraid to ask questions that might sound silly. Don't be afraid to ask—be afraid of what you don't know, or what you failed to find out.

When we had picked Dr. Pokorny's brain all that we could, we decided to discuss a possible date for the needle localization biopsy. The doctor sought to assure us that there was time to make this convenient for us. "It doesn't have to be done immediately, but I would not wait several months to do it." Pressed for more direction in this decision, he offered this observation: "Since we've found this questionable site early, I feel very comfortable in waiting as much as two months before proceeding to the next step." We had been planning to leave in two days for our annual vacation to Cocoa Beach, Florida. Our plans were to go by way of Tennessee to visit Karen's dad who was currently in a nursing home recovering from neck surgery. We decided to stick to our plans and try to enjoy a few weeks out of town, not surrendering our plans to the whims of an undiagnosed threat.

Here Karen and I misread each other's intentions for the first time in this crisis. She assumed that the kids and I were looking forward to getting out of town for a while. I assumed that she also wanted to get away and think about what was ahead for both of us. Karen and I discussed this, but we tiptoed our way around each other's feelings instead of speaking frankly to each other. She decided that it would be in everybody's best interest to postpone the surgery until we came back off vacation. We met with the appointment secretary and scheduled her needle localization surgery for August 11 at Baptist East Hospital in Louisville.

We informed our children about the scheduled surgery and told them we were still leaving on our vacation as scheduled. All of us were very eager to spend a few days together without duties and appointments, without homework, telephones…just plain getting away from everybody. When you live in a small town and operate a funeral home, the job can be especially demanding. It's hard to get away from the job. People often believe they can talk business with you at the grocery store, ballpark, church and anywhere they see you. So this little vacation offered our family some valuable privacy and quality time. Little did I realize there would be a stranger riding with us, demanding our attention and barging into our family.

Before we left on vacation, Karen and I wanted to confer face-to-face with our family physicians, Drs. David Jones and William Voskuhl. On the day before we left for Florida I called his office early in the day to see if we might visit with them at the end of the workday. Dr. William Voskuhl agreed to meet with us. His nurse said she would call us when the doctor was nearly finished with his patients and we could come on in to the office at that time. We met at the office about 6 PM and sat out in the empty waiting room—just the three of us talking.

I gave him a copy of the written document Dr. Pokorny had given us about this cancer. Dr. Voskuhl looked it over while we described the course of action Dr. Pokorny had recommended to us. I asked our doctor for his opinion and he concurred with Dr. Pokorny.

I then sought a means to assess the danger we were in. "Doctor Voskuhl, if, God forbid, this happened to your wife Debbie, how worried would you be about the future?"

He frowned thoughtfully and considered his feelings before answering. "I believe I would be concerned but not worried. This seems to be, at worst, a small cancer and very treatable."

Karen then took her turn. "Doctor, we were planning to take our regular vacation to Florida for the next three weeks. Do you think it is a good idea for us to go on vacation at this time? Or do you recommend that we stay home and begin treating this immediately?" He told us to go ahead and leave and have a good time.

We left for Florida by way of Tennessee, driving along the route we usually take. From our house it's about 900 miles to Cocoa Beach. Adding the additional mileage required to stop and see Karen's father, the trip totaled nearly 1200 miles. We drove the 300 hundred miles to Tennessee on the first day and the rest of the way the second. All that time in the driver's seat gave me plenty of time to think about our current situation and the prospects for the future. Too much time, as a matter of fact.

This stranger called 'cancer' takes over your thought process and makes it difficult to relax. I found myself driving down the road almost in a mindless daze, my mind constantly sinking into the worst possible thoughts. I felt like my wheels were caught in a rut, pulling my car into the ditch. My wife and I stared silently ahead for long stretches of time, both of us deep in thoughts we didn't choose to share. We found ourselves being a little short-tempered with our children. It was hard for me to concentrate on anything other than Karen's possible cancer.

Mileage markers sailed by, and I barely noticed the passing of time from deep within this gloom. Apparently my silence was appreciated in the back seat, though. We were almost all the way to Cocoa Beach when one of the kids exclaimed, "Dad didn't hardly complained about the music we were listening to like he usually does." Apparently I had remained too distracted to be my typical grumpy self. This stranger riding with us had demanded all of my attention and taken away time I always enjoy with my family.

The standard Grayson family vacation doesn't involve a lot of day trips and activities. When we go to Florida, we like to do nothing but rest and relax by the pool or on the beach during the day. In the evenings, we usually go out to eat and then find something the kids want to do. Standard selections in this category include the go-cart track, batting cage, or the putt-putt course. We usually try to catch a matinee movie when the afternoon storms come. Every other year or so we will try to tour the Kennedy Space Center or drive back into Orlando for a day at some of the many theme parks. But doing nothing tops our agenda.

Once we arrived at our condo, our spirits naturally picked up. Just being together on the beach without the usual daily hassles improved our emotional state. But that stranger didn't stay away for long. Afternoons spent reclining in the Florida sun didn't seem as peaceful as I remembered them to be. Peace and quiet gave my mind the chance to wander back to our health situation.

I noticed that Karen was less interested in our evening activities than usual. The daily beach walks we have both enjoyed together each year barely interested her now. Perhaps she was feeling drained emotionally or physically tired. Either would have been quite understandable. Meanwhile, it became increasingly more difficult for me to do nothing. I felt as if I had to fill my waking hours with some sort of activity. I walked by myself, I cleaned the condo, I cooked and otherwise invented reasons to scurry around and distract myself. I needed to keep my mind busy doing something.

My wife and I just couldn't get on the same page. While I whizzed around like the white tornado, Karen wanted to do nothing. After we came in from the beach and supper was out of the way, she usually would lie on the couch and watch TV for hours at a time. The kids and I did most of the evening activities on our own, when she sank into this mood. I just couldn't get her interested.

On other days, she seemed to climb out of it. I remember all of us going to an afternoon movie one rainy day and we thoroughly enjoying the movie and our time together. The theater was located in the mall, which inspired some supplementary shopping. We drove into Orlando one day and visited SeaWorld. It rained and stormed almost the entire time we were there, but all of us enjoyed the outing. By the end of the day we were soaking wet and cold—a sorry bunch of Florida vacationers. On happy days like this, we hardly thought about our family health situation.

Despite bringing the whole family, Karen and I found plenty of time to share each other's company alone. After the kids went to bed, we usually played cards until late at night. We played rummy and kept a cumulative score for the entire trip. This particular trip I got my butt beat every night, to my wife's considerable satisfaction. Late evenings spent watching the moonlit surf from our balcony sitting provided us with important time together, and we took advantage of it.

In the thoughtful silence of that balcony, thoughts arose in my mind that I didn't dare to share. The unknown lay ahead of us, lurking over the dark waters of the sea. Will we ever know this type of peace and contentment again? What awaited us back home? Would we be able to vacation together again? Was this our last break before a steady increase of sickness and pain?

One night sitting on the balcony, Karen mentioned for the first time how nervous she was becoming. She interrupted the restful, rolling waves to air a thought that emerged from deep inside. "How difficult it is to face this without my mother." Karen lost her mother two years earlier, and that loss seemed fresh to her as she pondered the biggest crisis of her own life.

As our vacation began to wind down, the anxiety dug in. We knew what would happen as soon as we got home, and this impending pain made our trip home seem unbearable. Both of us faced our fears with a conscious effort to console each other. More and more of our conversations together centered on her upcoming surgery and the possible outcome, trying to cushion each other's fears from the impending impact of possible shocks. Hugs and handholding became more frequent, satisfying a mutual craving for comfort and contact. Just sitting together side by side in a restaurant seemed more important than eating. And just the desire to feel her touch was so important to me, in a manner of intensity I had never known before.

But no spin-doctor could make this thing go away, or put a positive twist on such a scary situation. It was very difficult for me to dwell on the positives. Hopeful platitudes seemed phony and insincere; they would not help. I knew I owed Karen my best effort to remain upbeat, but this new stranger would not let that happen. He stayed with me constantly.

With great reluctance we started the trip home. We decided to travel home a different way than usual, traveling up the East Coast of Florida and through South Carolina into Tennessee and then home. I believe we chose this route in order to delay our arrival home by another day. One more day away from home seemed to forestall the surgery a little more. Eventually, though, we came back home and settled back in. The van was unloaded, the clothes were washed and the house was cleaned before the surgery.

Vacation had given Karen and I the time to plan some strategy against this challenge. We wanted to face this new challenge together, as a team. Thus we felt it was important for us to meet with the doctors together and do everything together that we possibly could. Each of us had the need to be involved and the need to offer support to the other. The only way to provide for these needs was for us to experience as much of this challenge together as we possibly could.

This is exactly how we have lived our life together—sharing our experiences and responsibilities through equal involvement. Neither of us has specifically relegated responsibilities (such as 'she cooks the meals' or 'he pays the bills.') The mundane duties of cooking, cleaning, kids' homework and lawn mowing are all handled by both of us, in tandem, cooperatively. Ever since we met on December 27, 1975, we've tried to be there for each other.

We decided to attack this new hurdle facing us the same way we handled a hamper of dirty laundry or a yard full of leaves. As the spouse in this situation, I felt it was important for me to participate in everything I could. This involvement would give Karen encouragement and support, while serving as therapy for me. Yes, I had my own needs in all this. I needed support and comfort also, and the sense of usefulness in a crisis that comes from meaningful involvement. Up until this point, I had felt shunted to the sidelines in our biggest challenge. Karen was dealing with the possible cancer better than I was. As the day approached for her surgery, we decided that it was important for both of us to work this problem as a team.

On the day before the surgery, our emotions began to build and the tension between us grew. Those three weeks spent waiting for the surgery date had generated enough tension to build up a head of steam. We were in a state of uncertainty, allowing us to indulge in hurt feelings whenever the other didn't give the correct answer or facial expression. As a matter of fact, we had one of the biggest arguments we'd ever had. With less than twelve hours before surgery, we were arguing about things that were really not important. We should of been spending quality time together and supporting one another instead of fighting. Instead, we were both keyed up and unable to fall asleep, allowing all that built-up steam to escape in anger. Eventually we calmed down, felt a little foolish and acted civil toward each other once again. We finally got to sleep after midnight, certain that tomorrow would be a very difficult day.

On the way to the hospital I found myself trying to delay the inevitable. I was actually uncharacteristically patient on the highway, trying to drive a little bit below the speed limit. I definitely didn't want to get to the hospital any sooner than necessary. I have never believed in what some people call a nervous stomach, but this morning I most certainly had one.

We arrived at the hospital at the appointed time of 6:30 AM for a surgery that began at 9 AM. Anxiety was running high, the hands were sweating and the heart was pounding. But we wanted to tackle this problem together, and that meant I wasn't going to sit in the waiting room and hide behind an old copy of *Sports Illustrated* while my wife faced her crisis. Our plan was to work through this as a team and be supportive of each other. This meant that I would try to be with her at all times except during surgery.

We started at the registration desk, answering the same questions we did the day before when the hospital called to inquire about Karen's general health and whether she was allergic to any medicine. Then it was "sit and wait" for a doctor who would see us shortly. After the automatic 30-minute wait, they called Karen back. We both got up out of our seats and walked toward the nurse. She immediately stopped me, with the authoritative mannerisms of a traffic cop. "You may have a seat across the hall in the other waiting room and they will call you back when they are ready."

"Why am I not able to go with her now?"

The nurse responded with an air of certainty. "It is hospital policy. You will have to wait."

A little righteous indignation started to show under my collar. Just what were they going to do now that would prevent me from being with my wife?

The nurse remained firm in the face of such a nuisance. "They have to get her gown on her and put in a IV before you will be allowed back. This will take approximately 45 minutes and then you will be called back before she goes to surgery."

I felt that this situation called for a little common sense. "We've been married for 23 years and I have seen her naked before and I've given her shots before. Needles are not going to bother me in the least." I explained to the nurse that we had decided to remain together through all this, except for surgery.

The nurse showed no respect for such convictions. She rudely responded that policy prevented me from being with her. "Besides the room she is going to is not big enough to accommodate your wife, you and the nurse." She apparently thought that this doubtful afterthought would make me sit back down.

This was the first of many experiences I had with what has become that dreaded word 'policy.' Doctors and hospitals must, of course, focus their concern with the health of the patient. The patient has to be priority number one. But this emphasis does not demand a dismissal of the spouse. I am not merely an annoyance that needs to be swept aside—I have an active role in this unfolding drama, and should be allowed to do my part. It is all too easy to wave family members aside with an unexplained reference to 'policy,' whether or not such actions are warranted or conducive to the reassurance of the patient. There needs to be some pre-operative discussion with the hospital staff or a liaison to better understand the effects of their policy on the patient and his/her family.

This nurse's meager supply of patience was now exhausted. I was told quite rudely, "Go have a seat in the other waiting room." I decided against causing a big scene, but I was very upset. This hurt me very much. Maybe I was being childish because I didn't get to go with Karen when she went back. I don't know. I do know that being left behind while such an important procedure took place in the next room put me in the worst possible frame of mind. I was left to myself to wonder what they were doing in there, and I could only stew in my own emotions. Have they found anything out yet? How is Karen holding up? I was forced to endure this panicky uncertainty with blinders on, and it was almost more than I could handle. Maybe it is a male thing, but I felt that if I could be with Karen, I could protect her and make things just right.

I spent a long forty-five minutes reading articles out of magazines that I had no interest in. I sat by myself watching the flow of patients and their families coming and going out of the outpatient area. Loved ones watched and waited, their tension barely under control. Each announcement over the intercom brought anxiety to their faces. Medical personnel briskly moved about the room, navigating their way through all these frightened people and maintaining a demeanor of importance.

Doctors and nurses swarmed through the waiting room, briefing families about the condition of their loved ones. Each visitor waited nervously, fumbling through the same irrelevant magazines, listening helplessly while the doctor announced the fate of a loved one. The most dramatic moments of his or her life was played out in a public waiting room, in front of everyone else. It seemed unprofessional to me that doctors were unwilling to talk with the families privately. Their voices carried all over the waiting room, as they discussed matters that a funeral director would not allow to be overheard. This seemed callous and disrespectful to me. I hoped that our doctor would have the decency to discuss our situation in private.

I waited nervously for the call to join my wife. Finally the waiting room receptionist called for me to come forward to her desk. I jumped up, knowing that I would now be allowed to be with her before the doctors began. But the receptionist surprised me by announcing: "They have taken your wife down and she will return in another forty-five minutes." I immediately thought they had begun the surgery before I was able to see her again. I expressed my displeasure with this. The receptionist now sought to reassure me, saying, "They have only taken her down for the needle localization part of her surgery."

Needle localization involves a needle inserted into the breast in the area of the tumor. The purpose is for the needle to guide the surgeon to the appropriate area for the biopsy. No one had mentioned that she had to go down to the X-ray Department to have this needle inserted before surgery. These omissions and contradictions simply increased my raging anxieties, adding to the impression that I didn't need to know what they were up to and that policy was designed to prevent me from finding out.

I was very upset at this change. In addition to the inevitable worrying, I had to make room for guilt feelings from not being around to comfort my wife. In fact, I was so upset at this time that I left the hospital and went directly to my van and began to write. Sometimes when I'm really upset, I write in a notebook for therapy. This writing usually vents some frustration in words not legible to anyone but me. I scribbled and sputtered for almost the entire forty-five minutes before calming down enough to return to the waiting room.

They finally called me to the front desk and a hospital volunteer showed me to the room where my wife was waiting. As soon as I got to her room, I noticed that there was space enough to accommodate our request to be together while they were getting her undressed and the IV inserted. In fact, we could have invited a few friends. I felt like I had been lied to and could no longer trust anything they told me. Karen shared my outrage and helped me to cool off.

My wife described what had transpired in my absence. The insertion of the needle apparently required no anesthetic, as none was used. Odd in this day of exorbitant hospital bills and high-budget medical technology that Karen awaited surgery with a needle sticking out of her breast and a modest styrofoam cup taped to her skin for protection. I was grateful that they hadn't attached it with duct tape.

An anesthesiologist and another nurse were making the rounds with all the pending surgery patients. They explained how Karen would be put to sleep and how she would feel after surgery. "We'll give you some medicine to calm you down, and then be ready for surgery in a few minutes."

The orderly arrived five minutes later to wheel her away. I kissed my wife and watched her ride away down the hall to face her ordeal alone. And I returned to my seat in the waiting room, to face this uncertainty with similar solitude. The two of us have stood together through every challenge of family life, and now, at our moment of greatest trial, we have been pried apart. I am told to wait patiently while someone else decides my family's safety and future happiness.

The pile of old magazines didn't interest me at all. Instead I began watching other families around me. They solemnly stared at the TV or magazine in front of them, concentrating on some vacant entertainment to distract their minds. Watches were frequently checked; every passing person in hospital white was carefully scrutinized for potential news of a loved one. We avoided eye contact with each other, knowing that each of us carried an emotional burden that deserved some privacy.

But privacy is an unachievable luxury in the waiting room, as it is in the hospital hallways. Intimate, painful matters were openly discussed, while the rest of us pretended not to hear. Once again I felt embarrassed for these other families. Symptoms were described, medical options detailed and choices were demanded regarding matters that were none of my business. It seems that patients and loved ones all must surrender their dignity before entering a medical facility.

The surgery lasted about one hour. I met with Dr. Pokorny immediately afterwards. He was thoughtful enough to save his commentary until he had taken me to a private area, a small room behind the receptionist's desk. There he invited me to sit and I stubbornly stood while he briefed me. "Everything went well. The incision was about 2 inches long. Upon opening up and examining the area, I went ahead and removed the entire mass, because it was only 5 mm. in size. Approximately 3 mm. of good tissue was removed in the area surrounding the mass. As before, I am unable to tell yet whether it is cancerous or not. But Karen tolerated the surgery fine and will be out into a room where you can join her in about 20 minutes." I noticed his effort to be precise and clinical, trying to reassure me with his air of honesty and efficiency. "I will call you on Saturday to let you all know what the pathology report shows." He rated the chances to be perhaps 80% to 20% against being cancer.

I received the usual instructions about how to bathe and treat the wound. "You should make an appointment in a week to remove the dressing and discuss any further options if needed."

It is at this point in the visit that some doctors stand impatiently and move toward the door, using a finalizing tone of voice to close the deal and move on to other duties. But I was able to ask Dr. Pokorny any follow-up questions about the surgery I could think of, and he took great pains to answer me thoroughly.

"Is this procedure also known as a lumpectomy instead of a needle localization biopsy, since you went ahead and removed the entire mass?" I was interested in this distinction for a variety of reasons. For one, I had waited under the assumption that Karen was getting a needle localization biopsy, and couldn't be present when a decision was made to change the strategy during surgery. Also, I was truly interested, after reading and studying about these tests and understanding a little of the differing implications of each procedure. On a more practical note, we had a cancer policy with our insurance company and I knew they would pay something on a lumpectomy. So I felt it was important to clarify this now and if the term 'lumpectomy' applied, get it documented now in order to avoid any trouble with the insurance company later.

"This procedure was in fact both, and I will document it as a lumpectomy on her chart."

I really appreciated Dr. Pokorny's willingness to discuss Karen's procedure and care with me in such detail. By showing such accessibility and openness, he made me feel that he had taken great care of Karen during surgery. In fact, we talked for a generous twenty minutes, without any feeling that I was detaining him or that he was rushing me out of his room. When we finished, the hospital volunteer directed me to a room. "Your wife will be here in just a few minutes."

Karen returned from the recovery room after surgery to this much smaller room. We were told that she would remain there until she felt ready to go home. This room was about a third smaller than the room she was in before surgery, the room too small for me to fit into. Various hospital personnel shuttled in and out of this room while my wife and I waited, and no one seemed to be inconvenienced by the tight quarters.

We headed home as soon as she was ready. Karen's recovery progressed as promised, with some soreness but no real problems. Discomfort around the incision made it difficult to use any muscles in her chest. She was not allowed to lift anything over 5 pounds and could only raise her arm above her head when she could tolerate the pain. For the first few days this meant she did not raise her arm at all. Bathing herself for the first week was difficult, as well as dressing each morning and undressing each evening.

Karen returned to work in a couple of days, well before recovery was complete. We both needed the reassurance of our normal routines to keep from dwelling on the diagnosis we expected to get on Saturday.

She refused to take any pain medication during the day while teaching, fearing that it would make her tired and not alert enough to function well. But she needed this medicine and took it each night and on the weekends, allowing her to get a good night's sleep.

Saturday came very slowly, bringing its verdict with stern deliberation. Weekends are busy in the funeral business, but I arranged my schedule so I could be at home when Dr. Pokorny called. That Saturday morning we were consumed with cleaning the house and catching up on the laundry, somewhat mundane duties to hold our attention at such a time. Without saying so, we both wanted everything in order in case our news brought a lot of friends and family to our door. Both of us now suspected the news might be bad, but neither admitted it to the other. The news might call for either celebration or consolation; either way it would attract a crowd of family and friends. At least the house would be clean.

When you have children in the house you never have to answer the phone. Our kids have friends who call almost constantly and our children jump up to answer the phone before the second ring. Ordinarily this is fine, but as the day grew later, our emotions began to churn with each incoming call. Each time the phone rang I held my breath and waited anxiously for the kids to yell for dad or mom to pick up the phone. So, after all this tense concentration on the phone, when the call finally did come from Dr. Pokorny, I was running the vacuum and didn't hear the ring. Karen answered the phone and told me to get on the extension so we both could hear the news together.

I immediately knew the news was bad. There was a clinical air of caution in his voice, an over-careful tone that proclaimed the seriousness of his news. I heard him say, "It was a malignant cancer, tubular in shape…" and my knees buckled. I just sank to the middle of the floor. The heaviest weight in the world pressed down on me, grinding me into the carpet, and I pounded my fist into the floor with wordless despair. I couldn't make out the solemn words now coming from the phone; nothing they said could help me now. Karen had to finish speaking with the doctor. He suggested that we get together next Thursday to discuss these findings and the next step in greater detail. In the meantime, if we had any questions we should feel free to call him.

But no doctor could answer the questions now roaring inside my mind. We both felt overwhelmed. I immediately went to our bedroom to lay down on the bed. Karen and I talked a couple of minutes and then I began to cry. I guess I kept it up for a long time. Karen had hardly ever seen me do this in 23 years of marriage, but if I had been waiting for a good reason, now I had one. The tears were unstoppable, a rushing flood from an overburdened soul. At this point, Karen had to take the role of comforter to keep me from falling into deeper despair.

Karen had been a smoker for over 20 years. In the back of my mind I had always suspected that somewhere in the future we would face lung cancer together. This breast cancer, at her young age, was totally unexpected. I couldn't believe that cancer had invaded our house so early, when so much of our hoped-for happiness was yet to come.

Anger and fear rushed though my mind. Predictably, I raged at God for our painful plight. What had we done to deserve this? What justification or greater good could come from such a cruel verdict? It just didn't make any sense.

As a funeral director, I am conditioned to expect only the worse. After all, those uplifting survival stories never cross my desk. Instead I have seen more than my share of undeserved consequences and unhappy endings. My mind turned too easily to the worst and tortured me with the morbid details of any potentially unpleasant scenario.

Unanswerable questions raged inside my head. How would she adjust to chemotherapy? How bad would she be burnt by the radiation treatment? How would Karen look and feel if she had to have a mastectomy? What would our future hold? How would this effect our lives? Would I be able to raise our kids by myself? Would I be able to help Michelle with her homework? I was simply swamped with self-pity, abandoned by any sense of hope, adrift in savage seas as I rode out the worst storm of my life.

Karen tried her best to pull me out of this gloom. She tugged at my arm as I lay sprawled across the bed and fought my depression with the best encouragement she could summon. "It's important to remember how fortunate we have been," she reminded me. "We were especially lucky to discover this so early. When that happens, the results are usually very good."

I couldn't manage much gratitude over the timing of this horrible news, so I shrugged off her hopeful words. This didn't stop her. "You can't tie yourself up with things that might happen. Right now we really don't know the future. We need to have some faith in God and adjust ourselves to this new problem. To speculate on it and expect the worst is just wrong."

"Well, then, I'm wrong to be worried, but that doesn't make it stop hurting."

Here was Karen, reeling from the biggest scare of her life, suddenly forced to put on a happy face because her husband was falling apart. This realization drove me into yet deeper despair. I wasn't interested in anyone cheering me up. This was the best opportunity of my life to feel sorry for myself, and I wasn't going to miss it.

When I had exhausted every encouraging word out of her, she let me drift through my gloom for a while. Eventually we both stretched out quietly on the bed, wallowing in wordless sorrow and clutching at each other. Time seemed to stop while we licked our wounds and shared some silent comfort. I slowly realized that my depression could only drag Karen down further. The pity party was over for me: it was time to swim back up to the surface and face the world.

My indulgence in depression had lasted about an hour—a tactical retreat from a reality I couldn't bear. There would be other such breakdowns, other moments when the gruesome consequences overwhelmed us. And there would be times when I was the comforter and

Karen remained inconsolable. But the worst of the shock wore off after a while and life came slowly back.

The room now seemed a little brighter in the late afternoon as we started talking again. It was time to face this, and to start by telling the people who cared for us. We discussed the sequence and procedure, how best to break the news to family and friends. Family love and a sense of duty finally pulled us off that bed and back into action.

We then washed off our faces, smoothed our clothes, re-made the bed and went to face our kids. They knew something was wrong, but they could only guess at the specifics. We told them the whole story. After they heard what the doctor had said, they left us quietly, knowing we needed our time together at this moment. They were very understanding. They went to their bedrooms and sadly watched TV until we were ready to go into greater detail and begin to deal with it all.

Family members had to be informed about all this. We collected ourselves enough to call Karen's brother Wesley. He and his wife Sandra were on the phone together when Karen explained to them what the doctor had said. She broke down and struggled to explain herself, until Wesley finally said he would call us back later in the day. We also called her other brother Charles and his wife Kay along with my parents and told them, and they, too, decided to get back with us later in the evening, when they had decided how they could help.

We then called our minister Rev. James Cash. He immediately joined in prayer with us and explained to us that everything would be all right if we just put it all in God's hands. Karen has always had faith in Brother Cash and I know she gets great comfort when he tells her everything is going to be okay.

Karen had previously needed and received the minister's consolation while her mother was a patient at the Vanderbilt Medical Center in Nashville. During the illness that led to her mother's death, Karen often mentioned to me how much she needed to talk with Brother Cash. We would then find a pay phone and call him and he would pray with her and she would always feel so much better because of it.

Karen has a strong belief in Brother Cash. She and I believe he is a true man of God and has been a great source of strength for both of us.

Karen decided that we needed to tell our neighbors Dewey and Sally Parker and Larry and Janet Bradshaw. They knew we were expecting a call from the doctor and we knew how concerned they were about Karen. We are very fortunate to have these two couples not only as neighbors but great friends. We know we can ask for their help any-time and they would do their best to help us out.

They were working out in the yard, so we decided to walk over and talk with them. They knew we were waiting for an important call, and apparently they could guess the quality of our news by the way we looked. Karen shared the medical details and answered their questions. But this type of cancer is so widespread that this news is liable to remind listeners of similar circumstances in others. Soon they share similar 'war stories.' Sally told us about her sister-in-law who had had breast cancer about 15 years ago. "She had part of her breast removed because of cancer and was left with a partial breast and she is doing great." I must have looked a little blankly at her, because she continued her explanation. "She had her surgery some 15 years ago and has done well. Medicine has advanced so much over the last several years and you will be just fine because of it."

We only stayed at our neighbors for just a few minutes before head-ing back home. We had talked ourselves out on this particular subject. By the time we walked home, our minister and his wife pulled into our driveway. He apparently sensed the need to follow-up our phone call with a face-to-face show of support. We visited outside around the pool and he reiterated to us that everything would be allright. After some heartfelt encouragement and prayer, they rose to leave and the next wave of well-wishers arrived. Sally brought her sister-in-law over for a visit with Karen.

After they left, Karen and I finally turned to each other and began mapping out a strategy. We discussed what the doctor had said and realized we were unsure of some particular details he had told us. I had become a frantic reader of everything I could find on the subject of cancer, determined to know as much about this cancer as the doctor knew. Now I needed more information: I just had to know exactly what kind of cancer this was. Since he invited calls with further questions, I called Dr. Pokorny's phone number and got the answering service. They called him and he called us right back.

"What is the medical name for this type of cancer?" I must have sounded like the meddling relative who second-guesses the professional opinion. But I hoped to spend time researching this type of cancer over the next few days. Then, when we met with Dr. Pokorny, we would understand better and be prepared to ask intelligent questions. A known adversary is less terrifying than an unknown, mysterious threat.

Dr. Pokorny must have understood my need to label and contain this cancer behind some specific terms, but he couldn't help but be vague about it. "This is just a tubular cancer. It has no real medical name." He fielded my next few questions and advised me to write down any further concerns as they come up and then bring the list with us to our appointment on Thursday.

This initially upset me. It felt like I had been brushed off; this doctor was relaxing at home and hoping to remain off-duty. My desperate mind demanded immediate answers, and couldn't wait until this man's weekend was over! It took me a while to get past this impatience, and to realize that he was right. Nothing would be decided right now, no matter how much I demanded it. As a funeral director in a small town, I knew how important your time at home is, and how you must defend it whenever possible. Besides, in my current emotional state, nothing the doctor told me could possibly give me any relief. The doctor was right to advise me to wait until the appointment.

The rest of that horrible day was spent getting back to family and friends, sharing details and accepting encouragement. We dwelt on the details of our crisis just as long as we could. We were emotionally exhausted, beaten down by this stranger between us. Routine household matters arose, but suddenly the interest level in them was no longer there. We both knew we must be strong for each other, but the mental strength necessary was just not there.

Finally, the day ended and we went to bed, although we talked for a while before trying to go to sleep. And we spent most of the night trying, with little success, to escape our worries and get some rest. I do believe Karen got more than I did. I tossed and turned most of the night and finally decided to get up about 4:30 in the morning. I tried to do some housework to keep my mind busy. I felt if I could work more I wouldn't be thinking as much about our situation. This didn't work for very long.

Over the next several days we had long conversations about what the future might hold. On Sunday afternoon we decided to get in the pool and relax and talk. We each got on a float and I laid my arm on Karen's stomach and we floated around the pool for two hours just talking and watching the clouds float slowly along. We felt some relief by remaining oblivious to what was going on around us. The phone, the neighbors and our kids left us alone. It was a totally relaxing experience; just what we both needed. In fact, we laid there so long we ended up getting sunburned.

Karen's brother Wesley called and we had a long talk. I suggested to them that it would be a nice gesture if they could come and be with Karen for awhile. Karen was stuck here in Indiana, a long way from her family. It might help her if someone would come and be here with her.

The anticipation of our next appointment was once again almost overwhelming. We wanted to hurry up and hear the final verdict; but then again, we weren't really sure we wanted to know. Because Dr. Pokorny couldn't give me a specific name or type of cancer, it was difficult for me to research and find out about this specific cancer that had invaded our household. I certainly tried to find out as much as I could about breast cancer. I spent countless hours on the Internet, where a great many sites offer information, advice and mutual support. There is so much information available and most all of it is written in easy to understand language. I also called the American Cancer Society at their number 1-800 For-Cancer. Within three days I had several booklets and brochures that were very helpful with questions and answers. I studied these brochures for several hours. I marked them up and compared their contents to information on the Internet, since it is not always clear how authoritative website information is. I also consulted our family physicians on several occasions. I even made a trip to the University of Louisville Medical School library with a family friend who had experienced the same thing. Cheryl Gilbert and her husband Richard were also a wealth of information. Richard and I spoke on several occasions about how he dealt with his experience and this gave me great insight as to what was ahead of us.

On Thursday, we grimly drove to the doctor's office to learn our fate. We had to stop at the hospital and pick up all of Karen's x-rays and films so we could see first hand exactly what the doctors saw. Once we had retrieved these from the X-ray department, we decided to open up the envelopes and examine the pictures before turning them over to the doctor. I thought I might be able to familiarize myself with the evidence here, therefore understanding more of the doctor's explanation. As we opened the folder to look at the films, we discovered that these pictures showed some other woman's breast surgery! Now we needed to return these films and try to figure out where Karen's films were. It took the x-ray department about fifteen minutes to find the correct films and we then proceeded on to Dr. Pokorny's office.

Dr. Pokorny examined Karen and appeared to be satisfied with all he saw. "Everything was progressing nicely," he declared. "After you get dressed, we will go to a room where we can look at the films together." Dr. Pokorny took the time to show us all the films and explain to us everything about them. He was very open with us and patient with my questions. He didn't rush us through to his conclusions nor did he refuse to answer any question completely.

On the wall were five or six x-rays lit up for examination and spread out for comparison. To our untrained eye, they all looked about the same. But a trained doctor looks for distinct signs and often knows where to look for them. Dr. Pokorny guided us to the area in question and explained why it was notable. It was indeed a tiny spot, but the tissue seemed a little denser than the surrounding tissue. Several small, cobweb-like lines extended out from this spot, like cracks on a sidewalk. "Without a previous mammogram to compare this with, I probably would not have identified this area," he noted. "All the inconvenience of scheduling annual mammograms and the discomfort of experiencing them…all that has now paid off for you. You have been very fortunate, and should consider yourselves lucky."

We then proceeded to his office, where we sat around a conference table. Dr. Pokorny left the room to get some brochures to help him explain exactly what type of cancer Karen had. He came back into the room and laid out before us three separate booklets about breast cancer. One was on breast cancer in general, another described the lumpectomy, and the final one concerned mastectomy. Immediately my eyes were drawn toward the booklet on mastectomy. I quickly felt sick to my stomach.

I had just finished reading David McCullough's best-selling biography *John Adams*. In the early 1800s, the President's daughter discovered a lump in her breast. The diagnosis today would be breast cancer, but the treatment back then was automatic: her doctors told her she needed an immediate mastectomy. Up until just 10 or 15 years ago, Karen's treatment would have been the same. Now, with regular check-ups and early detection, there are often less severe options.

But I wasn't thinking such positive thoughts at the time. I saw that booklet and I just knew that he was going to recommend a mastectomy. I braced myself for the shock of my life.

Instead, the doctor started off with a dramatic statement that I will never forget: "If my wife had to have breast cancer, this was the type of breast cancer I would go out and buy her." This immediately relieved the life-or-death pressure in the room and made us feel remarkably better.

Dr. Pokorny then went into great detail about breast cancer in general and the treatment that was usually done to combat it. His description was very precise and to the point but also very easy to understand. He explained how each part of the breast worked and this helped us ask what we thought were intelligent questions. He used the booklets and the diagrams in them and then also drew a few of his own. We have never had a doctor take so much time with us in describing a condition and possible treatment.

Prior to this appointment we thought it would be important for us to record our conversation with Dr. Pokorny. This would allow us to record everything correctly and also be able to double-check ourselves in case we disagreed on just what was mentioned. As everybody knows, two people don't always hear the same thing. This was our way of settling any disagreement we had about what was said.

"To understand breast cancer, we have to understand what the breast is, what cancer is and what are the specific characteristics of breast cancer." He began by describing the breast, a lecture topic I might have enjoyed more under other circumstances. "The tissue of the human breast is made up of glands called lobules that produce milk. Ducts extend from these lobules to the nipple, enabling mammals to feed their offspring. The remainder of the breast is fatty tissue, connective or lymphatic tissue.

"Cancers are actually an entire family of diseases that can cause any cells in the body to grow out of control. Although various cancers behave differently in different parts of the body, they share many common characteristics. Most types of cancer cells form a lump of mass called a tumor. The cancer is identified by the particular part of the body where this tumor first appears.

"Cancer of the breast begins in the tissue of the breast. Most of the tumors found on the breast are benign. They are abnormal but not at all cancerous, because they do not spread like cancer does.

"Other tumors in the breast can be cancerous but localized. These are called in situ, because they do not spread beyond the area where they appear. In situ breast cancers are confined to the ducts or lobules, and nearly all of these can be cured. Some oncologists do not consider lobular carcinoma to be a true cancer. But it can be an indicator of the potential for future and invasive cancers. This is another of the many reasons for regular mammograms to facilitate early detection.

"Finally, some breast cancers are invasive or infiltrating. These cancers appear in the ducts or lobules, but they begin to break down the duct or gland wall to invade the fatty tissue that surrounds it. These cancers spread in stages. In the local stage, it is limited to that area of the breast. Regional stage tumors have spread to surrounding tissue or nearby lymph nodes. Distant stage tumors have metastasized to other regions or organs. The seriousness of this invasive breast cancer is strongly influenced by what stage the cancer is in or how far it has spread at the point that it is first diagnosed."

The booklets he provided (and my own research) reveal the statistical horror of breast cancer. It is second only to the various skin cancers as the most common cancer in women, accounting for one-third of all diagnosed cancers in American women. In 1999, approximately 175,000 new cases of invasive breast cancer were diagnosed, along with nearly 40,000 additional cases of in situ breast cancer. It is the second leading cause of death in American women (behind lung cancer,) claiming the lives of 43,000 per year.

The risk of breast cancer increases with age for most women. This disease is uncommon under the age of 35, but all women 40 or older should consider themselves to be at risk. Most cases of breast cancer are identified in women over the age of 50 and the risk is especially high in women over 60. Research identifies several conditions as factors suggested an increased risk. These include:

- Personal history of breast cancer: women who have suffered previous breast cancers face an increased risk of recurrence.

- Genetic alterations: changes in certain genes make women more susceptible to breast cancer.

- Family history: a woman's risk for developing breast cancer increases if her mother, sister, daughter or any two or more other close relatives have a history of breast cancer, particularly if their case came at an early age.

- Certain breast changes: for example, atypical hyperplasia or lobular carcinoma in situ, or having two or more breast biopsies for other benign conditions

- Breast density: women aged 45 and over whose mammograms indicate at least 75 percent dense tissue are considered to be a higher risk.

- Radiation therapy: women whose breasts were exposed to radiation during childhood, particularly those treated with radiation for Hodgkin's disease. The younger the patient was during the therapy, the higher her risk to develop breast cancer in later life.

- Late childbearing: women who had their first child after the age of 30 have a greater risk of developing breast cancer.

The doctor detailed other potential indicators of greater risk. These indicators require regular check-ups: women who begin menstruation at an early age (before the age of 12;) women who experience menopause late in life (after age 55;) women who never have children; and women who took hormone replacement therapy or birth control pills over a long period of time. Each of these factors increases the amount of time their body was exposed to estrogen, making the later appearance of breast cancer more likely.

Then it was time to talk about Karen's possible treatment. "Just about everything is an option at this point," he said cautiously. "I would not recommend to us the use of chemotherapy, though. For this type of cancer, I believe that this would simply be overkill." For the same reasons, he did not recommend a mastectomy. But he did add this ominous comment: "A mastectomy is the only sure way to guarantee that the cancer would not come back in that breast." Nevertheless, he did not think it was necessary in Karen's case. "The prudent treatment for a patient of Karen's age and type of cancer is to treat it with radiation. And then, after the radiation is completed, the use of a medication called 'tomoxifin' will be needed everyday for five years. With the combination of these two treatments, her chances of its return will be less than 3%." I'm sure he has given patients much harsher odds than these, but he didn't make light of our situation. "There is still this chance of reoccurrence, you understand. But the odds will be pretty good against it."

So now we knew more about it, whether we wanted to or not. His lecture relieved both of us, and freed us from even worse suppositions. But Dr. Pokorny still had work to do. "We need to make sure the cancer has not spread anywhere else in the body. Breast cancer can potentially metastasize to the brain, bone, liver and lungs."

The stakes here were life and death. "It is vital to examine the lymph nodes," he explained with great gravity. "These are bean-shaped organs which are part of the lymphatic system." He thought it was imperative to prescribe a relatively new procedure called a 'sentinel lymph node biopsy.'

In other words, there will be more surgery. This dampened our sense of relief considerably. We listened as Dr. Pokorny again went into great detail about this relatively new surgery. "Just prior to surgery, Karen will be taken to the x-ray department and receive an injection of a small amount of radioactive dye directly into the breast. In fact, there will be four injections located at the corners of the previous incision around where the cancer was removed. The purpose of these injections is to make the lymph glands drain the breast of this radioactive material. As the lymph glands drain the breast, a Geiger counter will be used to locate which lymph nodes receive the waste material from the breast. The lymph nodes that drain the breast are located just under the armpit at about the region where hair begins to grow under the arm." Dr. Pokorny pointed to that spot and explained further. "Once the exact area of the lymph nodes is located, a small two inch incision will be made and the lymph nodes that were engorged with the dye will be removed. During the surgery we hope to remove somewhere between three and five lymph nodes.

"After removal, the nodes are sent off to pathology, where they are examined for any cancer cells. If no cancer cells are found, we will know the cancer has not spread to any other part of the body. If cancer cells are detected, then there is a greater chance that the cancer has spread to somewhere else in the body. If cancer cells are found, then Karen would be looking at a additional surgery and there would be a good chance she would need both chemotherapy and radiation." Dr. Pokorny did leave us with a hopeful assumption: "Because Karen's cancer is so small, I would be surprised if it has spread."

Our emotions blended mixed feelings of relief and apprehension. I have heard so many stories from families told by doctors after surgery that all the cancer had been removed, only to return almost immediately. This reoccurrence usually proved to be much worse than the original cancer. So my thoughts at this time were toward some of these families and their situations. I couldn't help wondering if we might be in the same situation.

I asked the doctor why he chose to prescribe the specific procedure he referred to as 'sentinel node biopsy surgery.' Some physicians share only their conclusions, without disclosing the reasoning behind them or the choices not taken. But Dr. Pokorny explained his recommendation. "This type of surgery is less invasive and also has less possible side effects. The other option is to do a more radical lymph node surgery called an 'auxiliary dissection.' This requires a much larger incision to remove all the lymph nodes in the underarm area. This procedure would increase the chances for more complications such as lympoedema, which causes the arm in question to swell tremendously. The patient is left with this for the rest of her life, along with a great loss of motion in the arm." We agreed that this was a gamble we'd prefer to avoid, but the doctor added this note of caution: "However, the sentinel lymph node biopsy may not work. In that case, you will have to make a decision whether or not you would want to proceed with auxillary dissection." The less invasive alternative seemed like a good place to start.

Doctor Pokorny pulled no punches with us. His frank disclosure of the various possible outcomes left the impression that he wasn't hiding anything from us. "There is a possibility that the sentinel lymph nodes we examine may be found positive for cancer. We will not know until several days after the procedure. If they test positive, then that would necessitate going back for a complete auxiliary dissection." But at this stage, under these particular circumstances, he regarded an initial auxiliary dissection as excessive. Surgeons now know from research that if the lymph nodes directly draining the area of the breast are cancer-free, then there is no need to remove any additional ones. You only need to remove those lymph nodes that are directly affected. If these first lymph nodes removed are not cancerous, then you know the cancer has not spread beyond that point. Why undergo more surgery than necessary?

Dr. Pokorny carefully described the upcoming procedures, to alleviate as much worry as possible. Even graphic details are appreciated, because the imagination can make an upcoming unknown far worse that it really is. "The radiologist will inject the breast with the small amount of technetium sulfur colloid, which is the radioactive substance we'll trace. Then the surgical procedure will take approximately an hour and a half and Karen will once again be put under a general anesthesia. This will also be done as an outpatient procedure. She will be able to go home as soon as she feels ready and is able to travel." We discussed the usual risks of anesthesia and the potential discomforts associated with this surgery, as well as the restrictions Karen must accept regarding movement and bathing in the days after surgery.

Happy to move away from worst-case scenarios, we discussed some of the implications if the nodes were cancer-free. The discussion turned to radiation therapy, its effects on the body and where the treatments might be needed.

Dr. Pokorny had mentioned that the sentinel lymph node biopsy was a new procedure, and this raised a few questions in my mind. "Approximately how many surgeries like this have you performed?"

His answer indicated some experience in this technique. He had performed about 20 biopsies, all but the first surgery he considered to have been successful. Knowing this made both of us comfortable in pursuing the surgery. Who wants to think of their surgeon struggling with some brand new, experimental procedure, scratching his head with confusion, burying his nose in some manual as he attempts to operate? "Medicine has made many advances in treating some cancers," he said with some pride, "and breast cancer is one of those cancers where gains have been made. Only ten years ago, if you had been diagnosed with this same cancer, the suggested treatment would have been a mastectomy. Now the patient has many more options to consider."

He gave us nearly two hours of his time, all of his pertinent knowledge and even some humor to relieve the tension he knew we felt. We decided to accept Dr. Pokorny's advice and proceed with the sentinel lymph node biopsy. It was still my intention to participate in every step of Karen's treatment, so I asked Dr. Pokorny what would be allowed. "Will I be able to go with Karen to radiology?"

His answer was cautious and professional. "I personally do not have a problem with your being there. But the final decision will be up to the radiologist."

I asked him to explain some of the hospital policies I had encountered during the first surgery. "The nurses were not willing to allow me to be with my wife at all times. Why wasn't I given the option of being with her during surgery?"

The doctor responded with frankness. "I personally don't care if you or one hundred other people are in the operating room. Your presence during surgery is not going to change how I perform the operation. The hospital is naturally concerned about any possible liability."

I could understand this, even though I certainly was not intending to sue anyone. But I still couldn't accept these arbitrary and unfair restrictions. "Why is it that when our three children were born in this same hospital, I was allowed to scrub up and gown up and be right there with her?" I was getting a little worked up, barely resisting the impulse to pace around the room. "There was much more exposed blood and body fluids when I was allowed to be with her. The procedure you are going to do makes only a small two-inch incision and there will hardly be any exposed blood. All I want to do is sit in the corner and be with my wife. I don't understand the difference in the two situations."

"I understand how you look at it," the doctor replied with considerable patience. "If my wife was having surgery, I would want to be there for her." I felt much better after explaining my side and how I was feeling. I think it has something to do with getting older and being stern in expressing how you feel.

Of course, none of this changed any of the "official policies" in place. Spouses were still regarded as unwanted, worthy only of exile to waiting rooms and sentenced to watch soap operas while their loved ones fought for their lives in the room next door. In the perfect world where hospital policy depended exclusively upon patients' welfare, I would have been encouraged to take a role and invited to come inside. I would have dressed up and scrubbed up just like the doctors and sat quietly in the corner of the operating room during surgery.

Perhaps hospital officials doubt that spouses can handle the emotional stress of such surgery. Yet the stress of being excluded, of being locked away from your loved one and kept in the dark about pressing medical matters seems at least as bad. And after all, I'm not at all squeamish about the hard facts of medicine and anatomy. I am an embalmer and funeral director; the blood, the odor and the atmosphere will not bother me. I couldn't get anyone else to understand this.

Dr. Pokorny shared his honest feelings on this matter, but he still had to defer to the authority of the radiologist and the smug policy of the hospital. He gave me the answer I knew he would give.

Karen's surgery date came upon us quickly. Karen's brother Wesley and his wife Sandra were going to drive up from their home in Tennessee to be with Karen and me. Karen enjoyed the support of visiting relatives, and they made me feel a lot better, too. I had denied myself this kind of support the first time around, as Karen pointed out to me. "You know, after the first surgery, our friends offered to stay at the hospital with us during surgery. But you drove them away."

"Now, just how did I do that?"

She was happy to explain it to me. I thought I was being generous at the time, because I just couldn't see any need for people to leave their jobs and homes, simply to spend time sitting around a hospital. I intended to reserve such inconvenience for myself alone. Instead, I managed to isolate both my wife and myself from emotional support during a crisis, and in doing so I also disregarded the concerns of those family members and friends who wanted to show their concern. Overall, Karen's assessment of my behavior on this point was not particularly positive.

I guess I should have known better. In my work I have enjoyed countless opportunities to watch families pull together to face crises and provide support. But my family has been different from most. The family business plays a large role in our relationships, and our work ethic dictates that "business comes first" most of the time. Furthermore, with two brothers and no sisters, outward displays of affection tend to be rare and awkward. This does not mean that we had no love or concern for each other. But after you work together ten to twelve hours a day, you need some separation. Otherwise your relationships will erode to that of business partners or co-workers rather than family members.

Consequently, we rarely take the opportunity to gather for a family meal or event. And when we do, our conversations turn inevitably toward the business, much to the displeasure of our wives. Perhaps this helps explain why I rejected our friends' attempt to stay with us at the hospital. As absorbed as I was in my overwhelming worries, I just didn't take the time to understand our friends' intentions. Karen helped me to appreciate that they meant well and felt the same urge to somehow help Karen withstand these challenges.

I got the picture. I dutifully apologized and, luckily, each of them understood my problem. They have remained very good friends. We must make considerable allowances for each other's eccentricities, especially during a family health crisis. And we should resist all urges to push our friends away at these times. Stoic suffering and stiff upper lips don't give us the strength we need to face such things.

The next round of surgery came up quickly. This time the surgery was scheduled for two o'clock, so we didn't have to be at the hospital until ten. Karen would have to suffer through that day, since she could not eat or drink after midnight the night before surgery. Missing a meal often gives her a headache, and she had enough hassles as it was. So we asked the doctors if it would be possible for her to maybe eat something at four or five in the morning instead of the usual ban after midnight. If surgery were scheduled for seven o'clock in the morning, she would need to endure only seven hours without food or water. If that was all right for that time frame, why would it not be all right for her to eat at even six o'clock a full eight hours before surgery? We were informed that they wanted to keep the patient without anything in her stomach because frequently there were changes in their schedules and she might go to surgery earlier in the day.

Wesley and Sandra planned to meet us at the hospital prior to Karen's surgery. We arrived at the hospital a few minutes after ten and registered at the outpatient desk. By now my wife and I felt like frequent fliers in this routine, but this familiarity did little to keep me calm. I still suffered the same nervousness and sweaty palms I endured through the first surgery. Once again I intended to participate throughout this whole procedure.

It was time to fill out the standard questionnaire about past medical history and medications Karen was currently taking. We gave them the same answers we had given over the phone the night before, when the hospital called us (I suppose to save us this trouble.) Don't they keep these papers somewhere? Within a few minutes, an older looking nurse with a deep voice announced that Karen Grayson should come with her.

We both stood up. The nurse immediately intercepted me. "Go have a seat in the other waiting room across the hall and when they were ready for you they will call you." Her tone was brisk and dismissive, as a mother might answer a child who asked to stay up an extra hour.

"Will I be allowed to go back and be with her while they get her ready for surgery?"

She decided it was necessary to repeat her previous instructions to me. With strained patience she explained why I had to wait somewhere else. "The room is not big enough for you with all the other people moving in and out. Hospital policy says you are not allowed at this time." The term 'hospital policy' was wielded like a trump card one simply couldn't dispute. She raised her voice a little to ensure my compliance. "We will call you when we are ready, and you may not come back until we call you." I had been squarely sent to my room.

Perhaps it was that matronly brand of command; perhaps it was the impeachable moral authority of 'hospital policy.' Either way, I submitted without an argument. I kissed my wife goodbye and Karen went with the nurse. I meekly took my assigned seat in the waiting room. I waited in the room nearest the receptionist station, busying myself by making a list of follow-up questions for Dr. Pokorny. Sitting next to the receptionist station provided me with a view of the elevators, so I could keep watch for Wesley and Sandra. I could also overhear the doctors as they discussed the condition of others that had just received some sort of treatment or tests. Why don't doctors have the common courtesy to speak to families in private?

I tried to focus on my list of questions, and time went by pretty quickly. In fact, after about forty-five minutes I became concerned that they might have forgotten about me. I decided to be nice and give them a few more minutes before asking what was taking so long. After about an hour of waiting I was called to the receptionist desk and another volunteer showed me to Karen's room.

"Where have you been?" was the irritated greeting my wife gave me. It seems the nurse who attended to Karen had called the receptionist desk about thirty minutes ago to ask me to come back. I hadn't come. Karen had then asked the nurse, "Would you please call the receptionist again to see where my husband is?" The nurse did call again and this time I received the message. We finally found out that when the nurse called the receptionist the first time, the receptionist had been all wrapped up in conversation with the other receptionist working with her. She forgot to call for me.

This time Karen was more upset this time than me. She knew they had called me and thought something must have gone wrong with me or that I had left the waiting area. Like I might choose this time to go see what was in the vending machines. I reassured her all I could. "You know I wouldn't leave the waiting room."

We finally got everything ironed out and Karen calmed down. "Have Wesley and Sandra arrived?"

"Not yet." Now she began to worry about them because she hoped to see them before surgery. Now she wondered if they were having some trouble. Didn't she realize that her own 'trouble' was more serious than anything we might manage on such short notice?

Within just a few minutes the anesthesiologist came in and spoke to us and explained how Karen would be anesthetized. This procedure would be very similar to the last surgery. The only difference was that she would be under for a little longer and it would take her just a little longer to wake up. Karen asked if he was going to insert a tube down her throat, because during the last surgery the doctors said they were not going to and after surgery her throat was sore for several days. He explained to us that they would not be inserting a tube. "The soreness you experienced had to do with the way you were breathing." After all our questions were answered, we waited for the orderly to take us to radiology for her injections just prior to surgery.

We had previously worked out a strategy for this. Instead of asking to go along with Karen at this time, I would just follow them. By doing so we hoped nothing would be said about hospital policy or anything to such regulation. When the orderly now arrived, he sat Karen in the wheel chair and we left for x-ray. When we arrived in the radiology department, Karen was the only patient waiting in the area. The orderly left us in the hallway while he went to tell them we were here. As soon as the radiologist came he took the wheel chair and spun Karen around. I was promptly excused: "Please have a seat in the waiting room and your wife will be out in just a little while."

I was expecting this and immediately protested. "I've received permission from Dr. Pokorny to be with her while these injections take place." His reaction was defensive and predictable. "Our hospital policy says that no one is permitted to go back with the patient." Just then Dr. Pokorny walked around the corner and I pleaded my case with him. They talked among themselves and Dr. Pokorny persuaded the radiologist that it was all right for me to be there. This ironclad policy appears to be negotiable after all.

Karen was placed on the table. After some small talk with Dr. Pokorny, he began giving Karen the injections one at a time. Once again Dr. Pokorny mentioned that they could not give her any Novocaine or anything else to kill the pain of the injections because that would interfere with the locating of the engorged lymph nodes.

As I had promised, I stood away from where they were working in order to stay out of their way. I did, however, manage to sneak a little toward the foot of the bed a little so I could see just exactly what was going on. Obviously Karen was experiencing a great deal of pain. I would think having an injection in your breast tissue would be much more painful that receiving one in the arm or behind. It looked like an effective form of torture.

He finished the injections quickly. I think Karen was a little more relaxed by having me with her. She even teased me a little bit about moving a couple of feet closer to the table where she was. After the radiologist checked everything again, we returned to her room to await surgery. We expected to wait about an hour before surgery could begin. This would give the radioactive material enough time to spread throughout the breast and the lymph nodes and thus make it easier to detect. Evidently, we were wrong, because within ten minutes they came to get Karen and take her away.

We kissed goodbye again and Karen was rolled into surgery. Once more I retreated to the large waiting room, assuming my usual position on a soft chair in the corner. The hands on my watch slowed to a painful crawl. Wesley and Sandra arrived in a frantic rush a half-hour later, and I briefed them on everything up to that point.

When I next checked my watch, ninety minutes had painfully passed. It was about time for surgery to be over; the anticipation rumbled inside me. The waiting room was filled with the bustle of a busy hospital—doors swinging open and closed, a steady stream of bedded patients wheeled past, people in masks and gowns examining charts and so on. The noisy paging of doctors formed a constant, annoying drone. Why do they bother to wear pagers when their calls are broadcast to the world? My legs twitched nervously and I tried not to check my watch too often. I wanted to get this over and get both of us out of there.

The receptionist suddenly broke this tension. "Your wife is out of surgery and Dr. Pokorny wants to speak to you." I eagerly followed her to a little conference room to wait for the doctor. Amidst my anxiety, I gladly noted that my doctor was offering me some privacy, and I appreciated the consideration. But time still dragged for me, and a few minutes seemed an unbearable wait.

By the time Dr. Pokorny arrived, I could scarcely control the tension I felt. "Everything has gone well," he announced. "We removed only two lymph nodes. There was a third area that I was uncertain whether it was a lymph node or not. Because I was unsure, I decided to remove it also. All the samples have been sent to the lab for examination." He then discussed Karen's immediate recovery. "The restrictions on movement of her arm will be very similar to the restrictions of her first surgery." Sadly, we were getting to be regulars on matters of this sort, and knew pretty much what to expect.

I summoned Wesley and Sandra and asked Dr. Pokorny to explain this surgery he just finished to them. He did so, adding a couple of details I didn't know about. "When she first went to sleep, we injected her breast with a dye that would help us in surgery to locate the lymph nodes that drain the breast. Even though we had previously injected the radioactive material, we still used a dye to help located the exact lymph nodes.

After injecting the dye, the breast must be massaged for approximately five minutes before the surgery can begin. This allows for good dissemination of the dye."

Boys being boys, I couldn't resist this topic. "I would have been more than happy to have performed this task. See? I told you there was a need for me to be in surgery with Karen." He chuckled without comment, perhaps preferring to reserve such perks for the professionals. Momentarily I pondered the duties of a therapeutic breast masseuse, until the doctor continued his explanation.

"When we inject this dye, it is possible for her breast to become stained by it. This may not clear up for several months. In such an event, it may be six to eight months before the tissue returns to normal." Dr. Pokorny then promised to call us on Monday afternoon or Tuesday morning to let us know what the tests revealed. After about twenty minutes of discussion and questions, I thanked the doctor and he left. Wesley, Sandra and I returned to the waiting room until Karen was released from the recovery room.

When she was ready, we were all invited to a room to see Karen. As before, this room was smaller than the room she was in prior to surgery—the one too small to allow me into. 'Hospital policy' appeared to permit these crowded conditions without a grumble. Karen was doing fine, and after about an hour she felt well enough to go home. We signed the necessary paperwork and headed for the door, hoping this would be her last surgery.

Wesley and Sandra followed us home and we spent the next couple of hours sitting by the pool talking. Throughout the next several hours it was my job to make sure Karen had an ice pack over her incision to prevent swelling and also to relieve some of the soreness. Our two youngest children were staying with our good friend Becky Zimmerman, who volunteered to entertain them for the day. Karen and I knew they were in good hands because they love going places and doing things with Becky. She treats them like royalty and this is just what kids want. Meanwhile, Karen needed a quiet house of her own.

Sandra fussed with Karen and Wesley distracted me; their presence took a lot of the tension away. Somehow we are taught to suffer our life's pains in silence and solitude, as much as possible. I'm glad to have outgrown this attitude and learned to accept the care my family and friends offer at times like this. Our friends have been very supportive and a huge source of strength for us. We know we would not have been able to get through this without their love and care.

It was getting past suppertime and few gut-wrenching dramas can prevent me from getting hungry. I told Karen that I would call out and get supper for everyone. As I played waitress and took the orders, Becky called. "My mother has cooked you a roast with potatoes and carrots and the works and a dessert. The only problem is that she doesn't have any way to get it to you. She's busy entertaining the kids and will not be able to get it to you until late."

It is a common gesture of consideration in Indiana for friends and neighbors to cater to each other in times of celebration or crisis. A wedding, funeral, illness or special honor is an invitation to covered dishes from all directions. It is a thoughtful way to help out and a personal and appreciated kindness.

I gallantly offered my services as a driver. Becky's mother and father, Clyde and Pauline Zimmerman, have been special friends of ours for a long time. I've had Pauline's roast once before and, believe me, it didn't take me very long to get to their house to pick it up. No bucket of fast food can match Pauline's roast. A good meal helped us shake off the tension of the day, and a piece of homemade cake helped make life feel good again. In fact, we each had a couple of pieces.

Wesley and Sandra returned home the next day and our household started to get back to normal. Karen knew she had stayed up too long when she came home from the hospital. Saturday found her in quite a bit of pain. She remained very tired for the next two days. "If had to do it over again," she admitted to me, "I would have come home and gone to bed instead of staying up and talking so much." Her body demanded the time it needed to recover.

Karen's arm movement was restricted by the pain and swelling. After we finished using the ice bags, I had to help Karen with her shower. She had temporarily lost feeling in her underarm area and this made it extremely difficult to shave and dress herself. But Karen refused to stay home from work on Monday, even though she was still in a great deal of pain. It was important for her to resume some sense of normalcy. Her dedication to her job was above what others expected. There were a few days immediately after surgery that she had to come home and rest before the school day was over. She tried to fight it, but the pain and fatigue were too much at first.

Your normal routine can be hard to find in an ongoing drama like this. Once again we faced the slow building tension of waiting for the phone to ring, bringing the important news we needed but dreaded. On Monday Karen arrived home a few minutes before I did. She checked the answering machine, and saw the light flashing ominously. When I got home she called me in the bedroom to listen to a message from Dr. Pokorny.

"Hello, this is Dr. Pokorny. I don't usually leave pathology reports on an answering machine. But since I have good news, I thought I would call you and leave a message if you were not home." My heart leaped to my throat, and Karen studied my face as I listened. "The reports have come back negative for cancer in the lymph nodes. This means you do not have to undergo any more surgery at this time. We are still waiting on the results of the keratin stain test to come back to be absolutely sure. We still need to get together this week. I will check over the incision then and we can talk over where to go from here."

Great news! I let out a yell of excitement. We embraced and kissed and then talked a few minutes before notifying our family and friends. Both of us felt more relief than we were willing to admit.

But Karen's body had been though a lot, and it didn't snap back into shape without some complaint. Over the next several days she struggled with pain and a lack of mobility in her arm. Sleeping was very uncomfortable for her and she had to use a pillow to support her arm. When she rolled over in the middle of the night I could hear her groan from soreness. All this tiring discomfort left her tired and very irritable. For a few days the kids and I had to watch what we said and what we did—a new challenge for all of us, I suppose, and one not immediately mastered. With the combination of lack of sleep, work and the pain, it was all too easy to attract the wrath of mom.

Over the next few days, any improvement was barely noticeable. Late that week we met with Dr. Pokorny again. He looked things over and approved, declaring "Everything is progressing nicely. The incision looks good." Those aggravating symptoms of pain and restricted movement were to be expected, and they would recede. He decided not to take off the butterfly strips over the incision, assuring us that these strips would come off by themselves over the next couple of weeks.

Karen asked about one small area that concerned her: the lower end of her incision under the arm. This area looked like a stitch remained hanging out after the incision was closed. We inquired about it because this little area rubbed up against Karen's bra and caused her a lot of pain. Dr. Pokorny affirmed that this was indeed a little stitch, and assured her it would go away in just a few days.

He directed our attention now toward the next phase. "Karen needs to continue with the next step of the treatment. This will be radiation of the breast to further decrease the chances of the cancer returning. Once you have had time to heal, which should be about four to six weeks, then it will be time to see a radiation oncologist for the radiation treatments." Gratefully, she did not have to rush into this next phase. "There is no great urgency in getting these treatments started, however. You should try to fully recover first."

I asked him, "Why wouldn't it be better to begin right away instead of waiting and allowing any leftover cancer cells to spread?" I guess I might have been showing a little more eagerness than Karen felt at the moment. But I wanted to be sure we were taking the most effective route to recovery.

The doctor explained himself in a steady, patient monotone. "This particular type cancer you have is a slow growing type. There is no cancer in the lymph nodes. When I removed the lump, we noted good, clean margins around the lump. This indicates to us that we have removed all the cancer. With the two surgeries you've just had, your body has been pretty worn down. Radiation will take a lot of energy from you. Since it is our belief that there is no more cancer, it is important for you to regain your strength before beginning radiation." This made perfect sense to us. This would also allow us to regain our emotional stability before approaching the next hurdle.

The doctor mapped out our upcoming maneuvers through the mysterious offices of various specialists. We had lots of new terms to learn. Before the radiation oncologist, we would need to see a medical oncologist. This specialist would be in charge of Karen's tamoxifen therapy. Dr. Pokorny asked us if we had a medical oncologist we wanted to go see. Thankfully we had never needed comparative shopping in this field. He suggested a medical oncologist by the name of Dr. Mitchell.

It all sounded reasonable, and the doctor's patient endurance of our questions helped secure our confidence. We agreed to go see Dr. Mitchell within the next couple of weeks and then we would return to see Dr. Pokorny again in his office. Then we would see the radiation oncologist, and perhaps continue working our way through the medical dictionary. Dr. Pokorny's nurse made the appointment for us and we returned home knowing we would have about a month to regain some control over our everyday life and get ourselves back to normal.

We had no idea what to expect from our visit to Dr. Mitchell's office. 'Tamoxifen therapy' is an impressive term, but it yields little meaning under careful examination. We didn't really understand why we needed to see this doctor. If he was merely going to look her over and prescribe some pill to take, why can't one of these other doctors do this? Will every specialist in the hospital get to take a turn on this case? I had to remind myself that our doctor's advice had been sensible and well explained. We should trust his expertise. We are not doctors ourselves (although we were beginning to talk like doctors) so we felt we needed to go hear what he had to say.

So we ventured into yet another medical office. Karen was given several papers to fill out and return. By this time we were proficient in recalling the information requested without having to look at medical and insurance cards. Redundancy has its rewards, I suppose. Within a few minutes we were summoned and shown to a room to wait for the doctor. Usually you assume your wait is over when they call your name, but often this is only the first step in an endurance contest. We waited about thirty minutes before Dr. Mitchell came in. He introduced himself and immediately asked us, "Why are you here to see me?" We had hoped that the files on his desk could have explained this. Karen answered simply, "We are here because we were referred by Dr. Pokorny regarding the use of tamoxifen after my breast cancer surgery."

He may have been relieved to hear that this wasn't a sales call. He asked numerous questions regarding Karen's cancer, and we tried to answer his questions as best we could. Eventually the conversation turned to the use of tamoxifen. Dr. Mitchell offered a simple explanation: "Breast tissue has numerous dimples. Tamoxifen is a hormone that fills in these dimpled areas and prevents estrogen from settling there. In doing so this helps prevent cancer cells from growing. Karen will need to take tamoxifen for five years. Because you are so young, there will be some discussion later in life about resuming this as a preventative treatment."

Dr. Mitchell then explained the risks of taking tamoxifen. "There is a chance of weight gain in the range of about ten to fifteen pounds on the average. Karen will immediately go into menopause, which usually consists of hot flashes and mood swings. There is also an increase chance of uterine cancer. Although this is a small chance, it needs to be followed by your gynecologist." Despite these sobering considerations, this is still the safest route to take.

We next discussed Karen's radiation therapy. Dr. Mitchell made a statement to us that weighed very heavy on our minds for some time. He said, "When radiation is given to the breast area, there is thirty times greater chance of lung cancer developing."

I reacted with some confusion. "You mean a thirty percent chance of getting lung cancer?"

He answered me quite sternly. "I mean thirty times greater chance of lung cancer."

I was shocked by these odds. "If that is true, then it makes no sense for us to proceed with radiation because the chance of breast cancer redeveloping is only three percent." Dr. Pokorny had not mentioned the chance that Karen might develop a new and serious cancer as a result of her treatment. I had not found this in any of my research either. This statement by Dr. Mitchell planted enormous doubt in our minds and caused us to rethink our entire approach to fighting breast cancer.

He shared further frank warnings. "When she is given radiation, there is no way to avoid the possibility of radiating a portion of the lung. The radiation oncologist will not tell you this, but it is true."

Here the advice of the varying specialists began to conflict with each other. When professionals differ in opinion, whom do you trust? While aiming for candor, Dr. Mitchell managed instead to plant the seed of worry in us. We had a deep trust in what Dr. Pokorny had told us from the beginning. Now we were unsure of what to do. I hated to doubt what Dr. Mitchell had just said, but someone was certainly wrong on this matter. Before we went to Dr. Mitchell, we were at peace with our plan of action. Now we just felt confused.

Dr. Mitchell prepared Karen for examination with brisk instructions. "Please disrobe from the top down and I will return in just a few minutes." He turned breezily and walked out into the hall. Karen put on the hospital gown while the doctor waited just outside the door. So we whispered to each to each other what we thought of Dr. Mitchell. Neither of us was impressed. I suppose some of his patients would defend him, but our impression was that he wasn't right for us. Sometimes when you meet people you can tell right away if you're going to get along. After this brief consultation with Dr. Mitchell, we knew we would not be back.

He reentered the room to commence the examination. His initial instructions were for Karen to open her hospital gown so he could look at her breasts. Perhaps this was routinely requested under the circumstances, but it immediately gave me the impression that all he wanted to do was to see her breasts. His 'examination' lacked clinical technique, and appeared to be simply aesthetic. Once he was satisfied with the view, he summarily closed her up and asked us to give him a call when she was ready to start taking the tomixfen. He would then write her a prescription. "There will be no need for you to see me again. Just call when the prescription runs out and I'll write another." Apparently a properly trained professional can inspect symptoms, diagnose an internal problem and prescribe an appropriate treatment simply with a casual glance at my wife's chest.

After our consultation with Dr. Mitchell, I felt a lot more confidence in our other doctors. He didn't have to tell us there would be no need to see him again: we had already decided this for ourselves. We both needed the advice of someone we could trust.

Although I felt irritated by this doctor's manner and actions, I didn't feel that I should immediately dismiss everything he had said. He did bring up the point about the radiation increasing the chances of lung cancer by thirty times. That was serious enough to demand further study on my part and an explanation on Dr. Pokorny's part.

Dr. Pokorny had also recommended a radiation oncologist named Dr. Janice London, who administered radiation treatment at the William F. Waller Cancer center in Louisville. His recommendation reassured us: "Dr. London is a patient-oriented doctor. If I or anyone in my family had to have radiation therapy, this is who I would go to see." Of course, this same doctor had recommended the dislikable Dr. Mitchell, but we decided to give Dr. London a chance. Dr. Pokorny's nurse made the initial appointment for us for the following week.

My wife has an admirable mental makeup that allows her to ride easily over the ups and downs of life. She accepts with equanimity all the cards that are dealt to her in life. She generally sails upright, looking for the best behind the clouds around her and remaining unruffled by the head winds. My ride is often rougher. While she resumed her routine of daily duties as teacher and mother, I continued my frantic research to educate myself on the next step of Karen's recovery. She may be willing to outwait her unkind fate, but I had to wrestle with it.

Still I was unsure how I should react to all this, or how I should feel. Does my alarm disturb her? Do my attempts to control my worries seem like I don't take it all as seriously as I should? What do my kids need from me to help them face this period of fear and uncertainty? At what point does my concern for my wife turn into pity for myself? Much has been written about caring for cancer patients, but few writers have bothered to help shore up sagging family members. A threatening and frightening illness effects every aspect of a relationship. I was sleeping somewhat better than a few weeks before, but still I was obsessing with the worst scenarios of cancer and Karen's condition. And even in moments of reassurance, the most morbid worries were never far away.

My research became my release, and I pursued knowledge with an unaccustomed thirst. If my college professors could see me now...! Perhaps I sought the empowerment of authoritative assurance, or perhaps I sought validation for my worst suspicions. Either way, I scoured the Internet for information that would help me understand what might lie ahead. While shopping with Karen and the kids at the malls, I haunted the bookstores and searched those shelves for information on breast cancer and radiation therapy. Somewhere I hoped to find the information that could beat this beast. I couldn't rest until I found it.

At home, I denied myself those habits that ordinarily relaxed me and distracted me from more ordinary concerns. Sports pages sat unopened while the coffee table gathered medical magazines and printouts from health websites. Always a passionate basketball fan, like any healthy Hoosier, I now found myself uninterested and unable to watch. Those who knew me well were shocked by this change.

My home was no longer a safe haven from life's troubles. We were never left alone. There was a stranger in my house that followed me everywhere I went. He demanded my attention and denied me any comfort. He hovered in every room, reminding me constantly that I have a lot to worry about and no time left to enjoy life. I've heard so many families that I've worked with tell me their loved one's cancer came back after they had hoped everything would be all right. This stranger made me doubt and dismiss every hopeful thought and concentrate always on the worst.

Was my passion for research helping me or hurting me? I now had a much better understanding of the situation before me, but an inescapable appreciation of the dangers. Karen and I talked one day about my problem with this stranger and my constant dwelling on the cancer. She tried bravely to penetrate my gloom. "There are scores of people in hospitals and nursing homes that would love to trade places with us. My cancer is very treatable," she reminded me. "According to Dr. Pokorny, I do not have any more cancer in my body. You just need to relax and get over it."

This blunt comment hit home, like a slap on a hysterical face. She was right. I was not doing her any good by constantly dwelling on the subject. She was the one with cancer and I was the one having all the problems. I couldn't help picking at the sores, as if I felt the need to match or exceed the pain she endured so bravely. But the caregiver and family members face different challenges than the patient does, and in some ways, it is harder for the loved one than for the afflicted one. When you are the patient, you have some degree of control over the situation. On the other hand when you are the caregiver, there is very little you can do or control. One is a participant; the other a bystander. I believe that, in my situation, the reluctance of the hospital staff to allow me to take a role or even to be with Karen led to my frustrated and rebellious attitude. Of course, I chose my own peculiar obsessions, but they helped drive me to them by trivializing my role to one of spectator.

As the day approached for our first appointment with Dr. London, the radiation oncologist, my emotions once again began to build. The quality of my work suffered, and so did the quality of time I spent with my family. I dreaded our first meeting with Doctor London and feared the vague force of radiation on Karen's body.

Naturally, I wondered how Karen would react to the amount of radiation she would be given. Would it make her sick? Would she become weak and or would she be burnt from the radiation? At each step on the progression of cancer treatment, we were exposed to war stories about other people's trials and tribulations with cancer. Now we heard more than our share of radiation nightmares. People mean well, but they can't help sharing stories that might better be saved for another time. "And you know what happened to her...?" These stories provided plenty of questions for me to ask our doctor. They also cost me a lot of needed sleep.

We arrived at the William F. Waller Cancer Center in Louisville at our appointed time. We immediately registered at the information desk and provided them the necessary information they requested. After completing the registration, we were told to proceed to the radiation area and present the nurse with the packet of paperwork provided by the registration clerk. Here we were again asked to fill out more paperwork and return it to the nurse. Bundles of data were shuttled back and forth, entered onto computer screens and stuffed into file folders. Every new patient requires reams of redundant documents.

We waited about fifteen minutes before being called back to an examination room to wait for the doctor. When we got to the examination room, Karen was asked to put on a hospital gown. A nurse then came in to ask several more questions and record the answers on yet another form. Many of these questions were now being asked for the third time in only thirty minutes. With all the lines now completed on her questionnaire, the nurse then proceeded to take Karen's blood pressure, pulse and temperature. We then waited a few more minutes until the doctor arrived.

Dr. London knocked at the door and came in to the room in a very pleasant mood. Accompanying her was someone we assumed was a resident doctor. Dr. London was approximately our age and appeared to be a doctor with a bubbling personality and a sense of humor. She opened with some small talk and then offered the same observation that Dr. Pokorny had said three weeks earlier. "This was a good kind of cancer to have had." She emphasized the past tense. "You do not have cancer anymore. You are here as a preventative measure, and that's all."

She stressed the need for post-operative and preventative treatments: how important yearly mammograms and self-examinations would be for Karen. Karen told her she had not routinely practiced self-examinations before all this came up. Dr. London asked Karen if she had ever been shown the correct way of doing self-exams. Karen said not really and Dr. London promised her she would explain the procedure in great detail before she was released. The doctor then looked at me and told me it was important for me to know also. What's this? A role for the spectator? She said my involvement would make self-exams more interesting and probably more frequent.

"I'm more concerned about your smoking and the effects of that than your breast cancer." She offered a graphic description of the effects of smoking on the body. Like almost every smoker, Karen had heard this speech before and found the means to ignore it. It was my hope that now she would be willing to do something about it. Dr. London suggested that if Karen was truly interested in quitting, she could help her do so. She suggested being part of a study that at this time had a 97% success rate after two years. It involved medicine and nicotine patches. Karen would be on the medicine about three weeks before she stopped smoking and then use the patches for about six weeks. Karen decided to stop smoking with Dr. London's help, and they worked together on a plan of action.

Dr. London then explained how to proceed with the radiation treatment. "After you have healed from your surgery, which is usually about a month, we will have you come back in and get set up for the treatments. At this appointment we will be taking numerous x-rays from different angles and you will be given a CT scan of the torso. After studying the results of the x-rays and CT scan, we will apply markings to your body which will be used to guide the technician when they give you your treatments." Dr. London suggested that Karen wear an old t-shirt on that day so the ink from the markings would not ruin any good clothing. "You will have twenty-three treatments that will be given 5 days a week. Looking at your skin tone, I would not expect you to have any of the burning and oozing of the skin that is commonly seen in patients with fair skin."

The unknown provides us with our greatest fears, so Dr. London then described how the treatments would actually be given. "You will lay down on a table and your right arm will be positioned over your head and placed into a guiding device. There will be a cone-shaped machine overhead and it will be positioned on the side of your breast and lined up with the markings. At this time a dose of radiation will be given and will last approximately 45 seconds." A pause permitted us to picture this. "The machine will then be positioned on the other side of your breast and the steps repeated. After the second dose of radiation, you will have completed your first treatment." She continued with some reassurance. "There will be no pain associated with any radiation treatment. There is usually some fatigue associated with radiation treatments, but research is inconclusive on whether it is caused by the radiation itself or by just having something else to squeeze into your life each day. You probably will have some redness and tenderness toward the end of the treatments and the breast sometimes can become firmer." The spectator quickly commented, "This might not be half bad after all." Karen then smacked me on the arm and told me to get my mind out of the gutter. I thought that Doctor Mitchell might insist on another exam, but I decided not to share this thought.

We continued talking about the treatments and some of the long-term expectations. Dr. London didn't back away from the cold facts of the matter. "If this cancer does come back after the use of radiation, the only thing do to at that point would be to have a mastectomy. The body can only withstand a certain amount of radiation in the same spot, and after these treatments you will have reached the limit. God forbid, if the cancer comes back somewhere else, you will be able to have radiation. But not on this breast."

Dr. London then took on the topic of tamoxifen. "You will need to take this medication every day for the next five years. There are some side effects, including going into immediate menopause, along with having hot flashes and mood swings. There is also a slight risk of uterine cancer." It's ironic, these cancer treatments that risk further cancers. Dr. London then turned to me and said, "Chris, the bad part for you will be while Karen is taking this medicine. She will be running around the house naked and because of her mood swings, you won't be able to do a thing about it."

"That's just my luck," I said. I wondered if I should warn the neighbors.

At this point, Karen and I both felt pretty comfortable with Doctor London. Her manner seemed open and honest, while her willingness to apply a little humor helped break the tension. We looked at each other and I could tell Karen was happy with the idea of having the treatments here at the William F. Waller Cancer Center. Having the patient's confidence encourages the patient's cooperation and this does a lot to ensure the effectiveness of treatment.

We then informed Dr. London of our desire to fight this cancer as a team.

When Dr. Pokorny recommended surgery for Karen, he suggested Baptist Hospital East in Louisville. At that time, we didn't think to investigate how to ensure that I would have a role in this battle. We took Dr. Pokorny's word and had faith that our request would be satisfied. Clearly that strategy had not been successful.

This time we decided to investigate everything ahead of time. What will the Waller Cancer Center allow? What will not be allowed? We did not feel obligated to have Karen's treatment at this particular treatment center—perhaps we should shop around for an institution that respects our wishes.

We told Dr. London how important it was for both of us to be able go through this together. Both of us were concerned here: both of us were effected, and both of us needed to be involved. I told Dr. London, "It is important to both Karen and me that you and this treatment center permit us to fight this battle together." I explained how this cancer was affecting my emotional stability and how difficult it has been for me to be brushed aside by doctors, nurses and hospitals. "This has created great emotional stress on Karen and myself. What makes it so terrible is that it could all have been avoided if there had been better communication between us and the healthcare officials before we started battling this cancer."

Now we have learned from our mistakes. We decided to talk up front with doctors, hospitals and treatment centers so as to avoid any additional stress on us. If one institution insists on its policy of needlessly quarantining those who care, we would find another facility.

Doctor London promised to respect all of our wishes to the best of her ability. She did insist on one rule: "When Karen is actually given her radiation no one is allowed in the room with her."

I accepted this restriction. "I understand this. But I would like to be with her at all other times if possible."

With these matters now behind us, we next considered when Karen should begin her treatments. Dr. London suggested toward the middle of September. Karen stated, "I would like to wait until after my birthday to begin."

"When is your birthday?"

"The 20th of September."

Dr. London checked her calendar, stating, "I always like to begin the set-up process. This is where you come in for your markings and measurements on a Friday and then begin the treatments on the following Monday." Karen checked her appointment book and everything was clear for Friday September 25th. We made an appointment for 2 o'clock on the 25th and were told we would be there about and hour and a half.

Mark and LaDonna Johnson are good friends of ours who live in Charlestown and operate an insurance business. They are approximately the same age as Karen and I. A couple of years ago Mark was diagnosed with Hodgkin's lymphoma. He underwent chemotherapy once and radiation twice and is doing just fine now. Karen and I had talked with them several times regarding Mark's progress during his treatments. As friends we were genuinely concerned for them. But naturally we were also interested in any information applicable to Karen's case.

Mark and LaDonna have been a tremendous source of information for Karen and me. Now that Karen was getting ready to undergo radiation, my mind drifted back to some of the conversations LaDonna and I had regarding Mark's treatment. Mark and LaDonna were trying to battle Mark's cancer together, just like we were. I can remember LaDonna telling me, "You have to stand up for what you want and don't take 'no' for an answer." Her advice displayed some of the forcefulness she has no doubt wielded in a few waiting rooms. "Not only are you fighting cancer, but it seems you also have to fight the doctors, nurses and hospitals, and this is not right."

LaDonna related an incident that demonstrated how she coped with reluctant healthcare personnel. "At one time the nurses told me I couldn't go with Mark and be in the same room with him. I turned around and told them I was going to and you had better not try to stop me." No muscle-bound bouncer appeared to evict her from the premises. She told me squarely, "You have to demand what you want and then turn around and fight for it."

We asked them what the radiation treatment had been like, and they agreed with practically everything we had read on the subject. "Sometimes you will be tired toward the end of the radiation," Mark explained, "and maybe a little tan and tender, depending on your skin tone." There was no mention of some of the things related to us in those worrisome war stories.

"How do the doctors actually put the markings on your chest?"

"I decided to get tattooed so I didn't have any of the ink marks," said Mark. "This worked better for me and you can't even see the tattoos."

This was the first time I had ever heard of being tattooed for medical purposes. I immediately thought of the type of tattoos you see on so many people today: how would Karen look with a large bull's eye on her breast, or some Allen Iverson artwork? Mark explained, "These tattoos are just small points of ink about the size of a pin head. It is a permanent mark and it only hurts just a little bit." I immediately decided to do everything possible to convince Karen not to get tattooed. I just couldn't imagine seeing her for the rest of her life with these permanent marks on her chest. It would be a constant reminder of what we had been through and I just didn't want her to have them. Perhaps I was being a little selfish here, but I was also being intimately honest.

But I'm not the only one in my family who believed in painful honesty. My mother served some up for me one evening at our home. We were all relaxing by the pool when I started complaining about the usual medical matters. I was, as usual, consumed with the emotional burdens of this cancer battle. Adrift in righteous indignation, I shared my thoughts on a long list of painful matters, from voyeuristic doctors to clinics that hire bouncers to maintain order. It's been reported that I ranted just a little and perhaps repeated some previous performances. When my mother could stand to hear no more, she stepped up and let me have it.

"Will you stop it? Will you stop these pitiful obsessions of yours? We all know how much you care for Karen and want to help her, but this is NOT helping. Karen has enough on her mind without you putting on a scene in public."

Her opening volley had been brisk and loud. I assumed the proper stance in such circumstances: shoulders stooped, chin to the chest, throwing myself on the mercy of the court. I think my mother surprised herself by the force of her outburst. She toned down a little, but her words to me were no less urgent. "As a mother and as a mother-in-law, I thought carefully about how I could help you two in this time of need. I confined myself to prayer and to being available as a sounding board when you needed to vent your feelings. You know that I don't mean to interfere. But increasingly I've been concerned that you are becoming compulsive in all this. The constant research, as if only you can save her; the unending criticism of doctors, nurses, hospitals, and anyone else who tries to help her...Just listen to yourself."

Close families give you the opportunity to relive the formative events of your childhood again and again and again. Right now I was a teenager once more, just rebellious enough to push my limits, but still attached enough to feel the pain when I was reprimanded. My mother and I reprised our roles perfectly.

"You want to show everyone how much you care; how much you've learned about the subject; how devoted you are by attending these treatments with Karen. You keep telling us how rude they were to you; how misleading they were to you; how offended you were. It's all about YOU."

I waited for someone to object, but no volunteers stepped forth. "Some counseling would help you, Chris. The stress you feel is very, very real and you can't help carrying on like this. But Karen needs more from you than this. She needs for you to be strong and support her, and not to weigh her down even more. She needs for you to accept what is happening. You cannot fix this; you cannot make this thing go away. Have faith, like your wife has faith; it will come out for the best."

I then dared to peak at Karen, and saw that she was smiling at me. I hadn't seen her do that very often lately.

Funny, isn't it? A funeral director, who needs to show compassion to the suffering in his work every day, losing his way when dealing with his own family's health crisis. Caught up in the personal fear and pain, I had lost sight of the things that were most important. I was outraged, offended that this cancer could barge into my world and shake it so hard. I was frustrated by something dangerous that I couldn't control.

In short, I had been way too human lately, and I knew that that wasn't good enough. I always offered more to my clients. Now it was time to give my wife and family some of that same consideration.

Who but a mother could make a speech like that? Who but a son would take it?

Karen began to feel better over the next several days. Her soreness and limited reach above her head was almost gone by now. She could once again bathe and dress herself normally. She did have one small area of pain along the incision of the sentinel lymph node biopsy. This was due to a little stitch that was sticking out of the lower end of the incision and was very painful when touched. The pain was compounded because this stitch was located just at the right level where Karen's bra rubbed it. Needless to say this made it very uncomfortable to wear a bra for any length of time. This was usually the first thing Karen removed when she got home from school. Dr. Pokorny assured us that this pain would go away after it heals.

It seems that the older we grow together, the less our birthdays and anniversaries mean to us. Our birthday celebrations have waned over the years, perhaps as the increasing years give new meaning to these milestones. But Karen had taken the effort to move the initial radiation appointment to a date after her birthday, so the occasion still meant something to her. Because of this cancer, I felt I needed to give her a surprise for her birthday.

After wondering what to do for several days, I decided upon desperate measures. An Elvis impersonator was booked to perform before her and the rest of the teaching staff at Northaven Elementary. I had arranged with the principal to schedule a staff meeting after school the day before Karen's birthday, when she would be least suspicious.

Elvis and I met in the parking lot (passing motorists must have wondered) and planned the deed. The principal smuggled him inside unseen and the King made a grand entrance into the library where this staff meeting was held. Karen was thoroughly surprised, embarrassed and amused. Hips swiveled, scarves were slung and swoons were offered up from the audience. The immortal Elvis sang several songs for Karen and presented her with a rose and birthday greeting, before slipping off toward future sightings elsewhere. I had accomplished my mission: to brighten the mood a little as we approached the radiation treatments.

All day on the 25th I was as nervous as I could be. Just the thought of having to start radiation treatments brought back most of the anxieties I had experienced earlier in our cancer fight. I left work and picked up Karen at school and we drove over to the Waller Cancer Center in Louisville. At least I knew I would be able to be with Karen, and this made me feel a little less helpless about it all. Since we had already addressed the situation with Dr. London about my need to be a part of the set-up and treatments, I knew we wouldn't have a problem.

We arrived on time and had to go downstairs to the radiation department. As we walked in we passed smokers standing on the outside of the building and outpatients leaving after receiving their treatment—clients and future clients. I could easily tell which were the cancer patients. Some were emaciated and wore wigs or turbans. Others were frail and needed help getting into their cars. Of course, these people could easily guess why we were here as well. I felt uncomfortably akin to these people—we shared some of the same worries and agonized over some of the same painful options. Even if the cancer has been completely removed, will it come back? Will we have to go through all this again sometime in the future? Will we look like some of this clinic's more obvious sufferers in the near future?

A quick registration at the nurses' station and a 15-minute wait preceded the calling of Karen's name. We both got up to meet the nurse who called us. We made it through the door together without any trouble. Karen had to stop and use the bathroom before proceeding, so the nurse and I exchanged small talk. It looked like I was going to participate in this phase, after all. Dr. London must have made sure the nurses knew of our desire to fight this together. I went through the door and everything was looking good.

Karen returned and we followed the nurse down a long hallway to where Karen was going to have the CT scan and the markings. When we approached the door, the nurse turned to me and assumed that breezy authority I had heard so many times now. She directed me to a seat down the hall and said that Karen would return in about forty-five minutes. Now, be a good boy and go sit over there...

Karen spoke up rather harshly before I even had a chance to complain. "We have spoken with Dr. London to get everything arranged so my husband will be able to stay with me during this time." She further explained how hard it was on both of us to be promised one thing and then told to do something totally different when the time came. Her tone of voice betrayed a subtle blend of exasperation and determination; an effective tone, no doubt mastered in the classroom.

But nurses get plenty of practice saying 'no,' and this one didn't back down a bit. "I know nothing about any such requests. Our hospital policy specifies that no one is allowed to be with the patient during this set-up phase." Out comes the trump card: any reference to a vague, undocumented 'policy' must silence all protest. Next up: the tired excuse that the room wasn't big enough for additional family members to be with the patient.

But we were battle-hardened by this point and refused to be turned away. Our nurse appeared to be thinking, "How come this isn't working?" She declared a tactical retreat: "Please just have a seat and I will page Dr. London to check on this. If she says it's okay, then you will be permitted to join your wife."

I soon suspected a bluff, but could do nothing about it. So I sat and fumed in the holding tank while Karen was taken away. I felt like I'd been sent to my room so the grown-ups could discuss something important. Here we had done everything we knew to do ahead of time to prevent this from happening and we still had trouble. Now Karen must face new fears all by herself while I wait pointlessly amidst a sedating assortment of old magazines and daytime TV. Primed by the tension of the occasion and insulted by this official arrogance, I was much too pissed to be helpful to anyone.

I could see the nurses and technicians beginning the tests and markings. I knew this because I could see the sign above the door telling everyone on the outside when x-rays were in use. I knew I'd been lied to once again. They told me they would page Dr. London, but now they were so eager to begin that they didn't wait for her to call back. My bloodstream boiled with waiting room rage.

After about 20 minutes Dr. London came down the hall and went into Karen's room. She didn't acknowledge me sitting in my little chair in the hallway, so I immediately thought I had been lied to by her, as well. But five minutes later she came and talked to me, hearing me out in my frustration and then taking me in to be with Karen

As soon as I entered the room and made eye contact with Karen, I knew something was wrong. Her face wore an expression I had not seen before, and I assumed that she too was outraged to see me plowed aside. I immediately noticed the room was indeed big enough to include me. The "small room" scenario must be a standard lie taught to nurses in training, to dispose of meddlesome loved ones. As our nurse had predicted, a lot of people moved in and out of the room while they set Karen up. But my presence caused no overcrowding or oxygen depletion; I wouldn't have interfered at all with what they were trying to do.

I stood out of the way while Dr. London explained what was going on. Karen lay on the table of the CT scanner and there was a machine directly above her. The lights constantly flicked off and then turned back on as they continued getting their markings. This machine projected lines on Karen's chest and two nurses with ink markers traced over these lines. This provided crosshairs for aiming, so the radiation technician would know just exactly where to position Karen during radiation. One worker recorded numbers as another read them from some sort of measuring device. They were measuring the area around the breast and also double-checking measurements taken with the help of the earlier x-rays. It seemed to me that everyone moved with brisk precision like experienced workers on an assembly line. There was little or no conversation with Karen on the part of the professionals standing around. Everyone was consumed with his or her task

Just before they proceeded with the CT scan, a nurse left Karen's side. He returned like a thief in the night to snap a picture of Karen. What a photo opportunity: she lay topless and exposed to the world with all these markings on her. This nurse said they had to have copies for the record. He claimed that this was necessary in case the markings ever came off, so they would know where to reapply them. He must have seen my skepticism. After using all of this high tech equipment to set everything up so precisely, would they have to rely on a couple of Polaroid pictures to reapply them? "Let's see here…begin about three inches below the shoulder…" No wonder the doctor spends so much time staring at the patient's file. Do they sit around the office at the end of the day comparing breast shots of their patients? I could just see them trading them like baseball cards, posting the best of them on bulletin boards and websites.

Once all the markings were drawn on Karen and all x-rays were completed, they proceeded to do the CT scan. I was able to watch as Dr. London looked at a television monitor and read out some measurements that helped them determine just where to aim the radiation. Dr. London mentioned to me that Karen's lungs and liver looked clear. I was especially glad to hear this. I have always been concerned about Karen's lungs ever since she had an echo-cardiogram done several years ago. During that test the technician asked Karen if she smoked and Karen said yes. She could tell from the image she had taken. The area around her heart looked cloudy, as she showed us. This was a result of smoking. Ever since then I have been deeply concerned.

After the CT scan Karen was allowed to get dressed so we could meet with Dr. London again before going home. We were instructed to wait for Dr. London in the hall so we could go over what would happen on Monday, the first day of the treatments. While waiting for Dr. London, Karen and I talked about how angry we both were. The same old lies added to an already stressful event. Dr. London joined us in about 10 minutes and began to explain that on Monday they would have to do some of the x-rays again to double check their measurements. If everything looked acceptable, Karen would be given her first treatment. We were told we would be there about forty-five minutes on Monday and then every session after would take about fifteen to twenty minutes. Dr. London promised that the technicians would work hard to keep everyone on schedule. She assured us yet again that I would be able to participate, just like we had been previously promised.

We then began to summarize our requests again and how important they were to us. We hit Dr. London with both barrels. We wanted to know if this was the way things would be going for the rest of the treatments. Dr. London assured us it wasn't. Even though she mentioned this to us, we were growing more skeptical with each visit.

On the way home our pent-up rage sought more immediate targets—each other. Karen had just endured a traumatic experience that had upset her and put her husband into a snit. I'm sure I could have been more attentive toward her feelings. But I felt like I was being slighted, and so I too quietly fumed with frustration. By early evening we had stopped talking. It remained quiet at our house through most of the weekend.

Karen examined herself in the mirror to see the full extent of the markings. Because she had been lying down at the treatment center she hadn't seen them yet. Now she did, and a look of despair took over her face. Ghoulish markings of purple ink branded her all over the front of her body, extending up her chest to the base of her neck. This prevented her from wearing any top cut below the chin, or everyone would be able to see this purple badge of illness.

We both agreed that these markings were unnecessarily extensive. I told her that I had seen the one male nurse getting a little carried away with his markers. He seemed to enjoy using his pen, like a frustrated body artist who couldn't accept clinical efficiency without a bit of flair. The infrared machine put out a narrow beam and the nurses marked along this line, primarily just to set the borders. Karen emerged with border marks outlining her breast along the superior and inferior borders and along with medial and lateral sides. It was the medial markings that seemed too much.

At this point Karen decided to take a shower. She decided to have me wash off the marking at the top so she would be able to wear more of her wardrobe. I also decided to wash off some of the other markings, leaving all the necessary markings for them to use. Otherwise, they could also consult the photos on their bulletin board.

I tried my best to play down the effect of these markings, which looked like chalk lines on slaughterhouse beef cattle, separating Porterhouse from T-bone. I couldn't believe she would have to look like this for the next five weeks. She wore a scarlet letter, a punishing reminder of the disease we were fighting. They assaulted her every morning from the bathroom mirror and lingered in her eyes long after the light went out each evening. Scars from surgery were not nearly so ominous or conspicuous or hard to take.

As the weekend progressed, our communication did not. We were still emotionally upset with the circumstances, the doctors, the kids and each other. In fact, on Saturday night I chose to sleep in our son's bed in his room in the basement. This was a response to being upset as well as being unable to sleep. She didn't need to be kept awake by my tossing and turning, so I figured I should sleep downstairs.

Still the sleep wouldn't come. I'd flop over and grumble a little, open my eyes to check the clock and see that only five minutes had passed since I last checked. Finally I dropped off around 3AM. I woke up late in the morning when I heard Karen stirring upstairs. I tossed and turned some more, trying to squeeze a little more rest out of the morning, and then Karen came to join me in our son's bed for a while. It seemed almost like a hotel room out-of-town. The kids were asleep upstairs and I didn't have to go to work (although I was on call and responsible for answering the funeral home phone.) So we lay alongside each other and talked once again. For the moment, no stranger sat between us. All those pains, frustrations and fears, so stifling that we had hardly spoken to each other for days, now relaxed to allow us some respite. We laughed and cried together for over three hours.

I retraced my feelings from the moment we found out about her cancer all the way to the present, and followed them toward the uncertain future. Some of these feelings surprised me as I explained them, as if I hadn't recognized them until I started talking them out. The more I talked about the situation the better I felt, even though the process was painful.

When I had finished pouring my heart out to her, Karen was sympathetic as always. But then it was time for me to gain some perspective: nothing I faced felt as frightening as what she went through every day. Karen was the one having to go through all the treatments, the embarrassing markings, the doctors' visits and the rest. It was Karen who had to learn to live with a potential threat growing deep inside her body. She had to find the strength to face this, and I had to do the same. Her stern advice to me was for me to get over it. "Accept it. Stop dwelling on the cancer and be more sympathetic to me instead of worrying about yourself. There is nothing that worrying will do but make you crazy. You cannot change anything about what has happened. So get over it." Even though this was difficult advice to implement, it was nonetheless true.

Now Karen opened up and poured out her true feelings about what she had been going through to this point. She mentioned, for example, how embarrassing it was for her to have to disrobe in front of everyone. It seemed that anyone in a medical gown had the license to look at, touch or squeeze her breast. This past Friday had been the worst of all. To be treated like a piece of meat instead of a human being was the most terrible feeling she had ever experienced. The curse of cancer removes all right to privacy and dignity.

"At least when I had my two surgeries," she reminded me, "I was exposed to the world only while I slept. I went into surgery with my clothes on and came out with my clothes on."

I could see how much this dehumanizing immodesty bothered Karen. The words flew out fast. "When I have seen Dr. Pokorny and Dr. London, it has always been in a private and professional manner. But then I get over there at the Waller Cancer Center and go for my markings and the first thing I have to do is undress in front of everyone. They lay me down on this small table and before I'm all the way down they begin issuing orders, yelling out numbers and they never say a word to me. They didn't even say hello, how are you or Mrs. Grayson this is what we will be doing to you. I look up and see three people are drawing on my chest, putting tape here and there, taking x-rays, raising me up and down, and moving me from side to side. The worst thing of all is when they are about finished, they quickly snap a few pictures of me and all the artwork they just drew. Can you realize how embarrassing this was? I was mad when I got in the room and twice as upset when I came out."

Some tears threatened to cloud her eyes, but her outrage drove them away. "I knew you were in the hall getting upset. I felt like I needed you the most, right then, but you weren't there. Then Dr. London comes in before she talks to you, and she is very cheerful like nothing is wrong. This made me more upset; at this time I was mad at everybody. I wanted to get out of there and I knew I had to go through with it. There was nothing I could do but lay there and feel humiliated. When I came home and looked in the mirror for the first time, I just fell to pieces."

Now the tears demanded their time. "It is terrible that I have to look like this for the next five weeks. I'm embarrassed for even you to see me like this. I still have a great many questions in my mind. How will I react to the radiation? Will I be burnt? How sore will I get? How tired will I be? How can I do everything I need to do at home and still teach? How accommodating will my principal be with me missing some school every day for the next several weeks? All of these things are going through my mind."

It was a mind packed under too much pressure. Karen told me she felt like she was having a nervous breakdown. I finally figured out a lot of her cold shoulder and unwillingness to talk is a direct result of this experience with the markings. The pressure and strain of under going two surgeries and trying to teach and not miss school has finally taken its toll.

It's a very uncomfortable comparison, but those who were shipped to concentration camps knew some of these same emotions. They were cruelly and deliberately de-humanized, in a manner surprisingly comparable to our treatment of cancer patients. Detainees were summarily stripped of their clothing, privacy and dignity, and rendered faceless by uniformity. They were made to feel unclean and hazardous, to be separated from healthy society. Identification numbers were branded on their bodies. They were torn away from their loved ones and assigned to humiliating duties. Uncaring guards ordered them around in a degrading manner. They were forced to carry on with their lives under unacceptable circumstances, without identity or family, without a shred dignity or hope for the future.

We both let our guards down a little that morning and shared the pain we had concealed inside. After talking all morning, we both felt better. There still wasn't much conversation over the next several days between us, but it wasn't withheld in anger or frustration. Now that we understood each other better, we allowed ourselves the space we needed to work things out.

On the morning of our first treatment, I lay in bed thinking of what I could do to help keep Karen feeling positive. I wanted to do something that would help Karen see her progress toward completion of her treatments. I had been cleaning out our downstairs office over the weekend and saw some of the silk flowers that Karen brought home from her mother's funeral. Just a few minutes before the alarm went off I had a brainstorm.

I went downstairs and counted 15 silk flowers. I needed 23, so I decided to have our local florist make an arrangement using these flowers and adding 8 others I would purchase. I wanted all 23 flowers put in a vase and delivered to Karen that morning at work. Karen would then take one flower out of the vase on each day of radiation. She would then take that flower with her to radiation and then put it in a vase I had placed in our living room. As the vase at school emptied out and the vase at home filled up, she could see her progress toward completion and recovery. I attached a note for Karen to read. It said that I knew she missed her mother; by using these flowers, maybe it would allow her mother to be with her each day as she went to radiation. It was a good idea—so good that I felt Karen's mother had inspired it.

Our appointment for our first radiation treatment was scheduled for 2 PM on Monday. I picked Karen up at school and we drove over to the cancer center. Once again my nerves stirred my stomach into disturbance. My hands were sweaty and cold, and I didn't trust myself enough to share my thoughts freely. Karen was more talkative, but nonetheless apprehensive about this first treatment.

We pulled into the parking lot and quickly went to the basement floor to the radiation department. After registering, we took our seat in a darkly lit waiting room with a huge fish tank and a large television set. You could hear the fish tank running and the television was on almost at full blast, but no one paid much attention to it. The walls were paneled and the carpet was dark brown—earth tones as sedative. I thought it was a particularly depressing atmosphere. Some brighter lights and more cheerful decorations might have helped the mood. The patients around us had enough to be depressed about already.

My wife and I tried to talk about anything but what we were there for. As people came and went I found myself wondering about the other people in the waiting room. Their faces were grim, the eyes cast downward in respect to my privacy and theirs. What kind of cancer did they have? How many treatments would they need? What war stories would they be too eager to share? The waiting room exhibited patients in the various stages of cancer. Some were very frail and old, broken down by cancer or perhaps by the efforts and extremes of treating it. Others were young and strong, not noticeably touched by the disease.

We were finally called back by the radiation therapist, who would check everything out and then give Karen her treatment. As we got back to the radiation area Karen was instructed to go the changing room across the hall and put on the usual hospital gown. I sat in a tiny waiting room and waited for Karen. When Karen came out of the changing room, I got up to meet her. She handed me her clothes and purse. It was my job to hold these for her. Having something like this to do was very important to me. It gave me a sense that I was needed for something. I know this sounds trivial and silly but it was one of the ways I needed to deal with this cancer.

We then walked around the corner to meet the therapist outside the radiation chamber. Karen stood in front of me at this point. The therapist very rudely asked me, "Just where are you going?"

Once again, Karen was quick on the draw. She explained that we had permission from Dr. London for me to be there. She explained what we wanted to do and why we wanted to do it. This made no impression on the therapist. We were once more instructed that hospital policy prohibits anyone but the patients themselves from entering. Once more the perils of overcrowding were described: "There will be several people moving in and out of the room and the room was not big enough for them to accommodate your wishes." She declared that all this was unheard-of. Husbands were never interested in being a part of their wife's treatment. Such concern was somehow unnatural.

"Well, I'm different," I huffed, "and this means a lot to both of us. We want to fight this cancer as a team." She then told me that I would have to go back to the small waiting room and wait for Karen. We tried to persuade her, but she stood firm, perched squarely on the righteous platform of hospital policy. I was stonewalled once again.

Thirty-five minutes passed before the therapist came to get me. I was outraged and demanded to know if Dr. London was here in the cancer center. If she was, I wanted to see her as soon as possible. I told the therapist we were not leaving until after we talked with her. She paged Dr. London and told me she would be here in just a few minutes. Karen quickly changed clothes while we waited for the doctor.

Now the therapist came by to explain that this hospital policy actually says only that no one could go back on the first treatment day. I would be permitted to go back the other twenty-four days of treatment. Aha! The ink was still wet on this policy. Immediately I wondered why they hadn't just said so up front. I now believed she was making it up as a cover story. An invisible document is easily amended. Maybe she thought I would drop my demands once I knew I had won the argument.

But she didn't know how annoyed I was. I was going to wait and have it out with the doctor, administration and any others who care to join in. We waited for about ten minutes for the doctor before Karen reminded me we needed to get back home because Michelle had a ballgame to go to. We talked a couple of minutes before deciding to see the doctor on our regularly scheduled day, which happened to be the next day.

As soon as I got to the car I had to let off some steam. I was about to explode. I screamed at the top of my lungs. Karen tried to calm me down and I, sadly, got mad at her instead. I just couldn't control myself. In retrospect it was a very selfish thing to do. But all this pressure just brings out the worst in us. I had been lied to and I didn't appreciate it one bit.

We returned home and got everybody ready for Michelle's basketball game. Karen and I didn't speak to each other a lot at that game. We sat down beside another player's mother, who just happened to be a nurse. She asked how the first day had gone and then wished she hadn't. We both unloaded on her. We told her the entire story about the visit to the cancer center from the first meeting with Dr. London through today's visit. She was shocked. She couldn't believe they acted that way, especially after they had told us we could proceed the way we wanted to. It made no sense to her. She said that patient care and the care of the family are equally important: often, patient recovery depends on the support of the family. A supportive role by loved ones is vital to the patient's wellbeing and necessary to the loved ones' emotional needs as well. After the game she asked us to keep her informed about how things went.

Before her first treatment, we asked if our appointment could be scheduled near the end of the day. We hoped to wait until after school, so Karen wouldn't have to miss any work. The lady who handled the appointments suggested that we take the first appointment of each day, at 7:30 AM. Karen is definitely not a morning person; she quickly rejected this idea. The lady at the desk assured us she would do her best to fit us in after school. It would be difficult to do because everybody else wanted to get treated after school or work. The only available time slot was 3 PM. Since we had no better choice, we decided to take it.

On Tuesday, I left work at about 2:15 so I could pick Karen up at school at 2:30. As soon as I drove to school, I noticed those familiar tensions kicking up. My stomach was churning once more, my palms were sweaty and I couldn't think of anything else but the ordeal we had to go through. My mind kept going back to what the radiation technician said before we left yesterday. Quoting, I assume from the hospital scripture, she had said, "You can go in with your wife on all of the other treatment days except the first." We would soon find out. Would a different shift and a new technician on the job bring about a change in hospital policy?

We turned down the street and saw a large sign proclaiming 'The Waller **Cancer** Treatment Center of Louisville' in bold lettering. Another greeted us in the parking lot with a perky 'Welcome to the Waller **Cancer** Center.' We pulled up to the gate allowing access to the parking area and saw a sign saying 'Parking for the Waller **Cancer** Center.' We pulled into a parking space and there just behind the parking bumper was a sign saying 'Parking for **Cancer** Patients Only.' On the front door, another sign read 'The Waller **Cancer** Center.' We rode the elevator down to the radiation department, looked up and discovered a sign directing us to the '**Cancer** Center' in the basement. As the elevator doors opened, we were greeted with another 'Welcome to the Waller **Cancer** Center.'

The word '**cancer**' was splattered everywhere! It struck Karen full in the face at least fifteen times as we walked from the car to the examination room. There was almost a hint of shame in this repeated proclamation. *"Abandon hope, all ye who enter…"* The word was the Scarlet Letter for all of us who sought treatment here. It was a label, a curse, the distinction meant to separate us from healthy society.

A nurse called us exactly at our appointed time. As usual, I went with Karen, wondering if further hassles awaited me. Would I be allowed to be with Karen or not? Had new passages of the Hospital Policy been handed down since yesterday? Karen quickly grabbed her gown and headed for the changing room to change. I stood in the hall for the minute or so she needed. She gave me her clothes to hold and we walked around the corner to face our fate.

We lucked out! Our technician was the one who was on duty yesterday. She made no reference to our skirmish the day before. We entered the room together. I was allowed in but instructed specifically where to stand. I saw that at least thirty people could have fit and worked in this room without cramping or collisions.

What a difficult job it has been to reach this simple understanding! How insistent had I needed to become to earn some acknowledgement of my role in all this! At least one technician in this place respects our feelings and wishes. Of course, all the others were still in doubt. Still, it was a relief to get past this silly battle for once and focus on the reason why I wanted to be here.

Karen moved through her newly learned routine. Lying down on the machine, as she had the day before, she swung her right arm above her head and into an armrest and guide. The technician turned the lights off and on in the room while she worked on positioning the patient. She even chatted a little with Karen. When she was ready, she told Karen to lay perfectly still and breath normally, two duties easily performed until we are instructed to do them. Then the rest of us stepped out of the room and the big door clanged shut. The technician stepped over to her computer and threw the switch to activate the radiation machine.

The technician's workstation sat behind a small office ledge that provided easy access to the instrumentation needed to administer the radiation. The work area had a little television monitor that showed Karen lying nice and still.

While running the radiation, the technician turned to me and apologized for yesterday's mix-up. No previous loved one had ever expressed interest in accompanying the patient. "I'm sure you want your wife to have the best care possible."

I said, "That's true, but having the opportunity to attack this cancer as a team is important to her care also." I guess I might appear dangerous to them, as some sort of opportunist cruising for a lawsuit and eager to catch them slipping up. This technician wanted me to hear her side of the story, but I was just as determined to let her hear my side. It was a standoff.

The first part of the treatment now ended. As the machine rotated to the other side, I stood far out of the way in the corner by the door. I didn't want to give her any reason to prohibit me from being there. After she got Karen re-positioned, we left the room again. I considered the worrisome fact that this radiation they were blasting my wife with was so dangerous that all others had to leave the room. Then I stood again at the desk and watched the monitor, waiting for our ordeal to end.

When the second treatment ended Karen got up and changed her clothes. We went to another room to see the doctor. We would see the doctor each Tuesday until the treatments were over. After a half an hour's wait, Dr. London came in. We had a long talk with her about yesterday's mix-up. She told us she was unaware of any policy that prohibited me from going with Karen on the first day.

"At least everything went fine today," Karen added reasonably.

"Good. Then hopefully we have all the bugs worked out so everything will go smoothly from here on out."

Karen then opened up discussion somewhat jokingly about my troubles dealing with all of this. She mentioned how I had lost my sense of humor and how I spent long periods of time dwelling on everything we were going through. Karen asked the doctor, "Is there something you could prescribe for my husband to help him through this time."

Now it was my turn to be scrutinized. Dr. London turned to me and asked, "Can you describe how you feel? When you are thinking so much about all these things, just exactly what are you thinking about?"

I told her I was spending a lot of time on the Internet trying to educate myself about breast cancer. "As an example, I wasn't satisfied when you told us Karen would have to undergo twenty-three radiation treatments. I had to know, why twenty-three? Why not fifteen or twenty? Thirty? I had to have a reason. Because no one had explained to me about the rads given and the total number you can have. I had to find out myself."

Dr. London answered me squarely. "Chris, I can go back to my office and get you numerous thick medical books to explain in medical terminology why twenty-three treatments are necessary for the type and size of your wife's cancer. You wouldn't be able to understand them, but trust me. There has been years of research to substantiate this number." Her tone was firm but professional. And then she turned the focus back on me. "If your time has been spent like this, you need some help."

I didn't have to wait long for Karen's reaction. She quickly said, "Thank God. And while you're at it, would you also give him something to help him sleep at night?"

I was analyzed a little longer and the doctor determined that it was important for me to be on some sort of medication for the short term. She said she would be willing to give me something to help if I wanted it. With a little encouragement from Karen, I agreed. Dr. London told me this medicine would take a few days before I felt any different. She gave us the prescriptions and we left for home, thinking things had been worked out to our satisfaction. Maybe I had been flying a little too low over the cuckoo's nest lately.

Or maybe the nurses had suggested that I be sedated.

When leaving the radiation area, you have to pick up a paper token to leave the parking lot without paying. As we picked up our token, we read the message on the back: 'Parking Token for the Waller **Cancer** Center.' A souvenir from this theme park for malignancy. We got back to the exit gate. On the arm that raises up as you leave were the words, 'Thank You, Waller **Cancer** Center.' I didn't appreciate all these subliminal reminders.

We were a lot friendlier to each other on the way home than we had been after the previous two sessions. Things would be a lot better now that we were finally able to tackle this cancer together. Our team approach was so logical to me that I couldn't believe that I was the first spouse or family member that wanted to be a part of the therapy.

All went well for Karen's treatment on Wednesday and Thursday of that week. We got in and out on time each day, which was important with our busy schedules. The more convenient we can make these things, the better we can buy into this treatment plan and make it work. The lady in charge of the appointment time told us on Thursday that she had an opening starting Friday at 4:20 PM. "Are you interested in this time slot? This would be your new appointment time for the rest of the treatments".

Karen grabbed it quickly. "This way I don't have to miss any school". This was even worth fighting the rush hour traffic home. Everything was going well.

On Friday Karen was scheduled for her fifth treatment. After today we could mark off one full week, with five silk flowers in the vase at home. We drove to the clinic at our new appointment time. While walking toward the radiology door, I noticed a new face on duty. She was a short, blond-headed nurse, talking with the nurse we had had before. Just as we got to the door, this new face immediately stepped in between Karen and me. Like a barroom bouncer, she got right up in my face and asked, "Just where do you think you're going"?

I said, "I'm going back to be with my wife, just like we've done for three days this week." I spoke just as bluntly as the situation demanded.

"No, you're not."

I cleverly came right back at her with, "Oh yes, I am." We followed this routine through a couple more times, until the topic seemed exhausted. Then I turned away and dared to walk into the room with my wife. The nurse protested very loudly and refused to permit the other technician to treat Karen until I left.

At this point I was really furious. I demanded to know how my presence with Karen interfered with the way they did their job. She refused to answer me. All she said was, "This is against hospital policy." She continued to cite this vague policy as if that word answered any objections and ended all argument.

The other technician, who had learned to be accommodating to us, never said a word as we squared off with the new one. I asked her a couple of times if I had interfered with her job in any way. The other nurse refused to allow her to answer my questions. She just kept saying it was not hospital "policy" for me to be there, with the same finality as "because Mommy says so."

Karen was now ready to boil over. She told all available personnel that we had been here for six different visits and we had been lied to on four of them. She refused to get on the table and decided immediately to have no further treatments at the Waller **Cancer** Center. If this was how they treated their patients, she wasn't going any further. She raised her voice and complained to the "boss lady" that I wasn't bothering anybody or anything. "In fact, it is a comfort to me to know he is here with me."

The comfort of the patient didn't seem to matter much. As before, the word 'policy' came up, as if it were some divinely crafted scripture unassailable by common sense.

I was simply shaking with rage and afraid I might say something I would later regret. But Karen spoke right up. "We are transferring everything to Lawson Memorial Hospital in southern Indiana". I suggested to her that she needed to go ahead and take today's treatment. After all, she was already here and dressed for the occasion. "Why not go ahead and get another one over with? If these people were so unqualified as to perform their duties with me standing and watching," (I turned briefly toward my listening audience,) "in violation of their own policy, then for today I will step out. We will speak to whoever is responsible for transferring records and get that started today before we leave."

I stepped out of the room and went to the desk, as I had done before. The childish "boss lady" even tried to cover up the television monitor so I couldn't see Karen. I didn't let her bother me. She then apologized to me, not for what had taken place but for the way it came about. She referred again to the ever-changing 'policy' and suggested I never should have been allowed to go back there in the first place. I told her we had followed what we thought were the proper channels, going through the doctor and discussing this from the beginning. "If we had known this was going to be such a huge problem for you to cope with, we would have looked elsewhere. It's that simple." I could tell she refused to allow herself to even consider our point of view.

I remembered what LaDonna Johnson had told me: "You have to be willing to stand your ground and fight with them and don't ever give up." This is what I was trying to do. I felt like I was trying to knock down a concrete wall with a rubber mallet. A fitting comparison, since I was getting nowhere.

After the first nurse got Karen set up and ready for her treatment, she disappeared without saying a word. This meant that the offended "boss lady" had to finish the job. Karen told me later that she didn't speak to her at all. Of course, she might have detected that Karen was in no mood to talk to her. When she returned to her desk, I continued to stand by it. She took a phone call from hospital security while I stood there. She told them everything was under control and they were not needed *(The on-call SWAT team now settled back down, relieved by the resolution of the hostage crisis in radiology.)* Hospital policy was safe for now.

Karen finished her treatment and walked out of the room. The self-important "boss lady" told us to have a nice day as we left, with a gloating tone in celebration of her victory. She informed us that we would have to see the appointment secretary to get all records transferred. I made her give me Dr. London's pager and office number. We had to let her know what had happened today. Out of courtesy to her, we wanted her informed immediately.

As I waited for Karen to change, the first nurse came down the hall toward me. I was still very upset as she came by. I asked if I could ask her a question.

She said, "Sure".

I said, "I see that you're pregnant and I wish you the best of luck. Is you husband going in with you when you deliver your baby?"

She said, "Yes he is."

"If at the last minute they came to him and said he wasn't allowed to go in with you, how would the two of you feel?"

There was a startled look on her face, betraying the thought of "no, that can't happen." She answered me, "We have talked it over with the doctor and everything is set to go."

I said, "Are you sure? Look what happened in our case right here."

"That would be terrible for us," she admitted.

Then I said, "Now you know just how I feel right now." She walked away without saying another word.

But hospital policies everywhere once banned husbands from maternity wards too. "It's too crowded for you to be in there—it would be too unsanitary—besides, no one else ever asked to stay with his wife. It simply isn't done. Now, be a good boy and wait over there until we call you." It took some patient assertiveness and family insistence to beat down that wall, and now husbands are encouraged to take whatever role suits them best in the delivery room. The benefits of mutual participation are now widely recognized in these situations.

Before we left, we tried to see the appointment secretary to get our records. The receptionist told us we would have to get permission from our doctor to release the records. We tried to call Dr. London as soon as we got to the car but the office was already closed. We were really just so upset we didn't know what to do.

The drive home was made a lot harder by what had just happened. I couldn't imagine any prescribed sedative that would have calmed me down. We talked all the way home about this bizarre situation. What had made them change their minds so abruptly? We couldn't figure it out. Was it something we had done wrong? What did they have to hide? We never found out what happened.

As soon as we got home, Karen called the doctor's office again to see if Dr. London was on call this weekend. The answering service said she was not and wouldn't give us her pager number. The only thing we could do now was to wait until Monday morning and call again. We called a few family and friends and told them what occurred. My face was probably posted by now at clinics across America: *"Likes to barge into radiation sessions; routine referrals to hospital policy are ineffective; should be considered dangerous and confined to waiting rooms."* No wonder they wanted to medicate me!

After dinner Karen took a nap. She had a slight headache and was totally exhausted. While Karen slept, I went out and sat around the pool to think things out. I had been out there about a half-hour when Mark and LaDonna Johnson stopped by. We wanted to talk to them about the doctor they had at Lawson Memorial Hospital. Did they like him? Were they pleased with his treatments and would they feel comfortable recommending them to us? They both said they would recommend them highly.

I asked LaDonna, "Do you think they would allow me to participate in Karen's treatment?"

She said, "They allowed me to and didn't seem to mind at all. They were very nice and cooperative. Just tell them up front what you want and they shouldn't give you any problems. You have to stand firm and don't take no for an answer." Both of them agreed that Dr. Carlisle was easy to talk to and get along with.

I told them how difficult the marking experience had been on Karen at the Waller Cancer Center. I explained one of the hardest parts for Karen has been dealing with the markings. Mark suggested having the tattoos done. I still wasn't crazy about that idea—I kept picturing a wife decorated like Dennis Rodman. I asked him if Dr. Carlisle did the markings in addition to the tattoos and he said he does, but he preferred to use the tattoos. Mark showed me the tattoos he received. When he pulled up his shirt I couldn't see anything. In fact, he couldn't find them either. He finally had to look at a small freckle on his arm to find something to make a comparison to. This changed my mind about the tattoos. If Karen could continue her treatments while not having to be constantly reminded of her situation with conspicuous markings, that would be great. I believed if Karen used the tattoos, she would feel more comfortable with the radiation. It would also allow her to have a greater selection of clothes to wear each day. It would be a relief to me, as well. I still wanted Karen to have the final say about which she preferred.

After Mark and LaDonna left, Karen got up and wanted to take a shower. What she really wanted was to wash off all those markings. I suggested she could wash a few of them off, but she really needed to keep the ones on the perimeter until we had seen Dr. Carlisle. If she washed all the markings off, she would have to undergo the CT scan and marking procedure again. If she left them on, there might be a chance she wouldn't need to do it all again.

Over the last couple of days of radiation, her breast and nipple became very sore. So sore, in fact, that it was hard for her to even wear her shirt. Before she took her shower she wanted me to look and see if see had sustained a cut of some sort. I could not see a cut or anything that would have caused her so much pain. It must have been the result of the radiation. We both thought that if she was so sore after only five treatments, by the end of radiation her pain would be horrible.

Another weekend was consumed with serious discussions on our present uncertainties and immediate future. Karen considered at some length abandoning her radiation treatments. At times she strongly opposed any further treatments, considering the discomfort and annoyance they had already caused, the potential for more serious side effects and their limited value. "Dr. Pokorny and Dr. London both stated that this therapy was merely a preventive measure," she argued. "They recommended that I take these treatments, but neither would try to change my mind if I chose to not take them."

She won my agreement easily on this matter: In my heart, I also wanted the treatment to stop and the aggravation to end entirely. But while my heart was saying to drop the trips to the clinic, my head was saying we must continue. I couldn't deny that I wanted to fight this cancer all the way to the end. I felt there would be no second chances. We had to do this right the first time, or forever regret our haste.

The unnecessary hassles with hospital staff almost pushed us into the hasty retreat. Both of us were very tired of being lied to. This extra stress put a heavy strain on our relationship. Each incident made me furious, and probably made me unpleasant company while I stewed. But to be treated as an intruder and shunted aside from a loved one who needed me was more than I could endure. Rather than offer my presence and support, I was dismissed, merely a chauffeur along for the ride. While pride played a part in my reaction, it was much more than just that. My sanity required that I take a role in her care. Karen understood where I was coming from: she was equally committed to our team strategy and equally offended by rudeness and lies.

The frustration affected my moods, and these added to our overall stress. Did Karen believe I was acting childishly at times? Probably…no, I know she thought so at times. In fact, in several of our heated arguments she offered that very observation. Did it hurt being told I was being childish, when I thought I was showing my concern? Sure it did, and this indignation drove me where I didn't want to go. On several occasions I decided that I would not go with her anymore. She knew where she was going; she could drive herself. There was no pain involved and nothing prevented her. What did she need me for? Clearly no one else thought I had any business at these sessions. In my cooler moments, I admitted that Karen's mental state might just improve if I stayed out of the way like the doctors and hospitals wanted.

But when the time came for Karen to go by herself, I found myself there with her anyway. I just couldn't bring myself to turn my back on her. Wasn't I fighting for the right to accompany her? Wasn't it because she needed me there and I needed to be there? Although we may have gotten mad at each other on several days and not talked to each other, I had to be there. A husband has to be there for his wife, and can't let pride or offense get in the way.

Karen called Dr. London on Monday morning to let her know exactly what happened on Friday. Dr. London had gotten wind of our skirmish and wanted to hear our side of the story. She got all the explanation she wanted from Karen in that phone call. Dr. London then promised that she would see what she could do, if anything. We wanted to know if she knew why this change in policy happened so suddenly. What had we done wrong?

Dr. London called back later that morning with the other side of the story. We were informed that the pregnant nurse said she felt threatened with my being there with Karen. "The nurse you had so much trouble with on Friday said that she couldn't do her job with Chris in the room."

Karen immediately answered this charge. "Chris didn't pose any threat to her in any manner. Furthermore, the nurse didn't mentioned anything to us on those three previous days he was in the room." She was amazed at how far this nurse was willing to go to defend her arbitrary behavior.

Finally, Dr. London laid it on the line. "Karen, the Cancer Center is not going to back down and allow your husband to be there for you. And since I work for the center, I have no choice but to abide by their rules. I understand what you want to do and why, but I am powerless to help beyond what I have already done."

We stuck to our guns too. The doctor agreed to help us find a new radiation oncologist and a center to have treatments. We told her we intended to finish treatments at Lawson Memorial and had hoped to see Dr. Carlisle. Dr. London said she knew Dr. Carlisle and would call him personally to fill him in on our wishes and the problems we'd had with the center. When asked if she could still be the doctor of record at Lawson Memorial, Dr. London explained that as a employee of the Waller Cancer Center she was not allowed to practice anywhere else.

Karen thanked her for trying to help and also for setting up our move to Dr. Carlisle. Karen said, "I hope you understand our problem is not with you but, with the treatment center."

Dr. London called Karen back later to inform her that she had spoken with Dr. Carlisle and scheduled our appointment with him for the following Tuesday morning. Karen's records and films would be sent over to Dr. Carlisle's office later this week.

We knew that switching treatment centers would extend the time it would take us to complete the treatments. I knew this would also be more difficult psychologically, just because it added more days to the task at hand. Some of the silk flowers would have to go back to school. We just wanted to get the whole ordeal over with and get back to the normal everyday life we'd lost a long time ago. But we both felt we had to take this route.

While we waited to see Dr. Carlisle, our life did settle back down. It was nice not having to go somewhere every afternoon; nice to take a few days off from a life-or-death drama. We came home and had dinner again as a family; we went to the kids' school activities together;

and, finally, we began enjoying each other's company once again. A burden had been lifted off our shoulders. Although we knew we had to start the entire procedure over again in a few days, I think it really help us out just to catch our breath after the mess we had at the Waller Cancer Center.

We arrived early for our appointment with Dr. Carlisle and went through the grim routine of registration. Still more paperwork to be filled out, but not nearly the piles of paper we had filled out at the Waller Center. We waited about thirty minutes before being called back to see the doctor. We spent this time watching television (at a normal volume) and reading a wide variety of magazines that dealt with issues other than cancer. Already we had noticed a great deal of difference in treatment centers.

A very personable nurse showed us to the examination room where we waited only a couple of minutes before Dr. Carlisle knocked on the door. We exchanged pleasantries and quickly got to the point of our visit. We summarized the last several months with Dr. Carlisle and why we were here to see him. I was carefully scrutinized—he'd probably seen my wanted poster. After looking over Karen's record, he reported that he hadn't received any films from the Waller Center. He had only received some written summaries from Dr. London that included all the marking numbers. He promised that he would make sure the omitted films were sent over to his office for review.

Dr. Carlisle then began describing how he would administer the markings and treatments. Much of this was a review to us, but there were some differences we liked. He said it would be impossible for him to use the same markings or measurements as the Waller Center. He described to us how precise these machines were and how important it was for Karen to be radiated only in the area that needed it. He wanted Karen to go through the marking procedure again to make absolutely sure of this. He recommended the use of tattoos instead of the markings, because they are more precise. He wanted to know if we had any objections to the tattoos.

Karen told him she would rather have the markings. She still wasn't comfortable with the idea of tattoos. I wasn't too keen on the idea myself until Mark showed his to me. If Karen had been with me that day, she'd probably feel differently about it. Dr. Carlisle suggested that we think it over some more. Perhaps we could start off with using the markings and then go from there.

I then decided to confront one of my biggest concerns. I told him of the conversation we had with Dr. Mitchell, the medical oncologist, and his confiding claim that radiation inevitably increases risk of lung cancer. Dr. Carlisle told us basically the same thing as Dr. Pokorny and Dr. London had said. I just felt more comfortable asking him like I did the other two. After he said what he did, we both relaxed and felt completely comfortable with continuing.

Dr. Carlisle wanted to know if Karen had any pain or discomfort from the five radiation treatments she had received. When she described the pain she felt around the nipple, he said he could block the nipple out so that area would not be radiated. It's not an area susceptible to cancer, so why cause women this irritation and pain when it is not necessary? There would still be a possibility of redness and soreness in the rest of the breast, though, as well as more firmness.

The doctor let us know that he had his own approach to radiation therapy. "I think we should also change the amount of radiation Karen is given just a little. The best method is to deliver less radiation to the patient at each visit and drag it out over a longer period of time. This lessens the chances of pain and soreness and also the erythema or redness sometimes associated with radiation." He thumbed through Karen's file and pulled out a chart. "Now, I see that at the Waller Center you were scheduled for 23 treatments of approximately 200 rads per treatment. Here you will be given 23 treatments at 180 rads. This will give you approximately 5000 total rads of radiation between both treatment centers." He further explained that radiation is accumulative and the pause between treatments wouldn't make a lot of difference to the treatment.

He peered at us over his glasses, evoking a little of the authority and charm of an old-fashioned country doctor. We had the impression that he held nothing back, and that we could trust his judgment. The doctor seemed to be both confident and open, willing to hear our concerns and explain everything in terms the patient can understand. We both felt very comfortable with Dr. Carlisle, and we were glad that Mark and LaDonna had recommended him.

When he finished his presentation, he asked if we had any questions. Here came the litmus test. I spoke up, saying, "Doctor, you've had a conversation with Dr. London and are somewhat familiar with the reason why we left her and the Waller Center." His nose dipped a little and those authoritative eyebrows emerged from behind his glasses. I told him of our friendship with Mark and LaDonna and he remembered her desire to be with Mark as he prepared to take his treatments. He immediately headed me off and agreed with our team approach. He even encouraged me to be a part of the treatment.

"Over my many years of practice, I have seen patients with no family involvement whatsoever. I believe the involvement of the family is an integral part of the patient's well-being and I encourage it whenever it is appropriate."

I appreciated these sentiments. But, frankly, I had been given more than my share of reasonable sentiments handed out by medical personnel lately. They cost nothing to give away and seem to do little good when it matters. "Can we then be assured by your authority that I will be allowed to be there with Karen?"

"There is a difference in the treatment centers," he responded with apparent candor. "Over there, they have many doctors, nurses and many policies. Those doctors each have to abide by their center's policies. Over here, I don't have a problem with you being with your wife. It's up to me, not them. I'm in charge."

"Will the nurses or technicians have a problem with me being there?"

There was a quiet firmness to his voice. "If I don't have a problem with it, neither will they. Do I make myself clear?"

I said, "Very clear." I'm sure that tone of voice was effectively deployed against nurses and technicians, as well.

He of course cautioned me that I could not be in the room while she was actually receiving each treatment. The technician must leave the room and duck behind protective shielding so as not to be exposed, and absolutely no one else can risk being in the room. I told him I understood that.

He told us he would schedule us Monday morning for the scan and then the measurements and markings a few days later. The treatments would begin as soon as they could be scheduled.

He'd said all the right things and assumed a posture that was both accommodating and commanding. We were reassured, although with reservations. After all, others had been just as reassuring. Time would tell and the Lawson Memorial Hospital would have the opportunity to prove themselves to us next week.

Through the last couple of weeks, our emotions had ridden a rough road. One moment everything felt good; then the next moment brought all sorts of turmoil. The medicine Dr. London gave me was just beginning to work. I'm wasn't spending as much time dwelling on our situation as before. My research continued, but that compulsive website stalking came to a halt. My interest continued, but my obsession faded.

Still, I never felt quite alone in our house. I relaxed better and slept some, but still sensed this stranger in my house. He faded into the background a little, but never went very far away.

Soon it was time for us to break in another medical clinic. We arrived at the Lawson Memorial Hospital for the CT scan. My typical symptoms returned: nervousness and sweaty palms. We went downstairs to the radiation office and were promptly sent back upstairs to the hospital's CT machine. There we met another lady who was also getting scanned today. The technician took us directly upstairs.

Things were very quiet on the elevator ride. I wondered if it would have been this quiet without me. Does my presence keep Karen from interacting with other patients? Karen and the other lady were shown where to change clothes. We stood in the hallway waiting for about thirty minutes while the other woman was treated.

Since we have sampled so many health care facilities lately, I couldn't resist studying my surroundings. This CT area was a little different from the Waller Center. For one thing, I didn't see the word 'cancer' written on every flat surface in sight. Here the monitors are located outside the room in a large foyer. We were too far away to see what was going on, but it looked like a good spot for me to watch the action when it was time for Karen's CT scan..

Then it was time for Karen to go. I was assigned to hold her clothes once again. As we both walked toward the technician, she immediately said,…Can you guess?

"Sir, you are not allowed to watch. I'm sorry, but it's hospital policy." I guess she decided to skip the stage where she claims the room is too small. Instead, she told me very nicely that I would have to return to the waiting room. "Your wife will be out in approximately fifteen minutes."

I didn't say anything at all. I just handed Karen her clothes and told her I would meet her in the car. I guess I'm the problem around here, I thought angrily. Apparently I'm holding up medical progress, taking up all that space and getting in the way of important people. While we stood waiting our turn, we noticed several people moving in and out of this foyer area. No hospital policy barred them.

These hospitals were treating me like an unwanted guest: someone crashing a party, a cheap thrill-seeker at a fire or auto accident, a pesky autograph seeker or some deranged celebrity stalker. Hospitals and nurses just didn't want me around. My own emotional investment in my wife's condition was irrelevant…I was merely a loiterer, a pest that needed to be shooed away like the family dog at dinnertime.

Karen returned to the car and we once again talked about the obstacles in our way. I decided to give them one last chance. I knew we had to come back for the measurements and markings in a couple of days.

The appointment for the markings was at 9 AM. We were hoping we didn't have to wait very long. The same technician who had performed the CT scan called for Karen to come back. As usual we both got up to go, and as usual…you got it.

"Have a seat, sir. Our policy says that no one is permitted back with the patient." This time she decided to add the one about the room not being big enough to accommodate our wishes. Hospitals everywhere must practice this routine.

Karen returned her fire. "Dr. Carlisle has given his permission for us to be together." She spoke with certainty, dismissing any objection, and maintained a much calmer manner than I could have managed.

This name-dropping failed to impress our stalwart technician. It took several minutes of persistent persuasion to make her back down. She let us by, but scowled with disapproval at this breach of security.

Then she led us into a very large room. It could've housed a major conference and sat one hundred people. She told Karen she would return in just a few minutes and while she was gone Karen needed to put on a hospital gown. She huffed on out of the room in a sizable snit. Karen and I looked at each other and agreed that she was going out to call the doctor, or perhaps 911. In about five minutes she returned, wearing the huge smile of the canary that had just tricked the cat. Now she smiled at us sweetly and was more than happy to accommodate our wishes. She must have gotten through to the doctor and gotten a clarification on her job description.

This procedure for measurement and markings was totally different here. The technician was the only other person in the room. No casual spectators or *paparazzi* photographers were in sight. Our technician explained everything she was doing to Karen in plain, understandable language. In fact, on several occasions she turned around to speak to me and see if I was following her explanation. When she was ready to x-ray Karen, we stepped out of the room. She even described to me the workings of the machine she was using and the reason the x-rays were needed. We repeated these x-rays again and once again she took considerable effort to keep me informed.

The topic of tattoos came up once again, and this technician also tried to persuade Karen to use them. "Of course, if you don't want the tattoos, that's okay. I just want to explain to you that these markings will be covered with clear tape so that the marks will not come off while showering." She told Karen how small the tattoos were and that she really would not be able to see them at all.

Karen finally waffled a little. She asked, "If I got the markings now, would I be able to change my mind later?"

"You sure can. And I'll bet that before we get too far into the treatments, you will decide to get tattooed instead."

Karen decided to think a little more about the tattoos and, meanwhile, to go ahead and get marked for now. We were finished in about ten minutes or so and ready to go home. We thanked our technician for being so professional with Karen during the whole procedure. I also thanked her for allowing me to participate and told her it greatly helped me in coping with our situation.

The next day the tape covering the markings started pulling at Karen quite uncomfortably. Bending and stretching was the biggest problem she had. Constrained and beleaguered, Karen hedged her bets further on these annoying markings. She decided to ask at the first treatment if it was okay for them to tattoo her in just one spot, so she could see what it was going to look like. She still wasn't sure about the tattoos, but she knew she didn't like the tape.

Our first treatment was scheduled for 12:40 PM on Thursday. We arrived and parked in the area set aside for radiation therapy patients. All signs directing us where to go mentioned nothing at all about cancer. Every sign indicated 'radiation therapy.' I know this is such a little thing, but it made a big impact on us. This was nowhere near as depressing as at the Waller Center. Even though we knew why we were there, it was important for us not to be reminded by the hospital everywhere we looked. There is certainly no shame in battling cancer, but it should be the patient's decision whether or not to proclaim an affliction in boldface lettering. This clinic's sensitive approach was appreciated.

We registered and were called back within ten minutes. I got up to go with Karen, a little shy of the potential crossfire, but this time I met no resistance at all. Still I felt like all eyes were upon me, wondering at my eccentricity and watching my every move. What was so weird about wanting to be with my wife? I definitely felt out of place. It was really a strange feeling. But even though I felt awkward, I knew I was where I needed to be.

We greeted the receptionists at the desk just inside the door. Walking away from them toward the radiation area, I could here them discussing me, as if I had created some sort of medical scandal. "He's the one who insisted on being here with his wife the other day. And he's going to be here each day as she does her treatments." Even though everyone was cordial and polite, I felt guilty for being there.

Climbing a small incline just outside the radiation room, we met the technician. She introduced herself in a professional manner and then explained everything to us once again. Karen was asked to step into the changing room and put on a hospital gown. While she did this, the technician laid out the ground rules for me. She said I would be permitted inside with Karen, but I must stand out of the way while she got situated. When it came time to give the radiation, everyone but Karen had to leave the room. After the first dose, we could go back into the room and the machine would be repositioned to give her the radiation from the other side. Again we would have to leave the room, but after this dose she could go home.

I briefly explained why I needed to be there for Karen and the technician understood my feelings and needs completely. She thought it was great that I wanted to be there. "This is just so unusual that it takes some getting use to."

Her openness made me more reasonable as well. "Well, I assure you I'm not here to look over your shoulders to make sure things were being done right. I'm not interested in suing anyone. I just need to be with Karen and that's all. After we get into this a little bit, I may just feel so much better that I might not have to come every day. Right now, though, it's important for me to be here."

This first session went fine; just like we had hoped it would go from the beginning. Karen came out with her gown on, handing me her clothes so I could do my job of holding them for her. The technician took us in the room and promptly introduced us to the other technician who would be working with her. My presence surprised her a little, but it was quickly explained. She also agreed that my request was unusual, but she seemed to be supportive. She explained to us there was one more person who worked part time with them and we could expect her to be helpful to us as well. Finally, she warned us that one visit per week would run just a few minutes longer because they needed to take some x-rays to monitor her situation.

Karen needed to get back to school right away. Driving back, we talked about how comforting this trip had been. They were true professionals in their approach to their patients. After only this first treatment we knew we had done what was best for us. We were very well satisfied.

I told Mark and LaDonna about our first experience with radiation at Lawson Memorial. They were glad to be kept informed. LaDonna made it a point to say how that facility's willingness to allow her to participate had helped her during Mark's treatment. Now that we have been through a treatment without having to fight our way through, I finally knew what she meant. Although we still had plenty of cause for concern, I no longer felt helpless and irrelevant in the care and protection of my wife.

After about a week of treatments, Karen asked if she could be moved from lunchtime to the first appointment of the day at 8 AM. The time away from school was beginning to bother her. Preserving her normal routine was important to her: she wanted to continue her treatment without interfering with her work. Even though Karen was not a morning person who climbed out of bed eagerly each day, she wanted to get her time changed. We figured she would only miss about forty-five minutes of school by going first thing in the morning, whereas the noon appointments consumed about an hour and a half.

Once we made the change to the mornings, things went even better. Yet despite our symbolic triumph and the validation of my husband's role, we weren't out of the woods yet. I still experienced the nervousness and sweaty palms each and everyday we went. We were still going for cancer treatments. There was no way of getting that out of my mind.

It was satisfying to see how personable these professionals were with every patient. They provided a friendly, supportive atmosphere that encouraged most of the patients to interact with each other. The waiting rooms became casual chat rooms where encouragement was offered and experiences were exchanged regarding their families, jobs and lives. The previous waiting room had felt like a holding tank for potential cancer victims: here we were people with lives, people preparing to survive and thrive. The difference was refreshing.

We gave our doctor a good report on all this and thanked him for allowing us to work together. I really think he appreciated hearing that from us. Then he got down to business, asking how Karen was tolerating her treatments so far. Was she having any problems with soreness, especially around the nipple? Karen told him everything was going just fine; although she felt considerably more tired than usual, she was otherwise okay. At least some of her fatigue came from changing our appointment time to the first one of the day.

But another matter was on my mind, and I found the opportunity to introduce the topic during our drive home. We were sharing our feelings of relief for catching this cancer as early as we did. "This could have been a lot worse," I suggested. Early detection saved us from dealing with a much more serious episode." Karen echoed these sentiments.

"I've been thinking that it's time now for me to get examined for prostate cancer." The passenger side became suddenly silent. "I can't help thinking that dad and his two brothers each had prostate cancer, and each of them decided to remove the prostate and cancer surgically."

Karen weighed my words carefully, examining them for deeper meaning. But I wasn't hiding any further suspicions. Dad and my two uncles have been monitoring their PSA (Prostate Specific Antigens) for years now, to detect any signs of trouble or recurrence. This simple procedure merely requires a blood sample every six months. I simply decided that it was time for me to determine my baseline PSA now. I seemed to remember hearing that men in their early 40s should consider this, in order to determine if troubles are developing later on.

My wife quickly agreed, and didn't miss the chance to remind me that she had been suggesting this for the last few years. My recent appreciation for early detection helped change my attitude, much to Karen's relief. I promised to line up an examination with the doctor who had treated my father.

When the time came for my appointment, Karen and I neatly reversed the roles we had played so many times lately. She rode shotgun alongside me and waited while I registered and endured the long list of inevitable questions about insurance and health history. Then we sat and waited. I imagined a simple blood test and a quick conference with the doctor. But as the nurse passed me a specimen cup, I realized that more was expected of me.

The nurse led us into an examination room and asked me why I was there. I reviewed my family history and my intention to start a monitoring routine, like a dutiful believer in precautionary testing. Nothing I said alarmed her; in fact, she said I was too young to bother about such worrisome things as PSAs. "We like our male patients to begin their blood work around the age of 50, in most cases." But since I was there anyway, she proceeded to draw some blood. Then she told us to wait for the doctor to call.

The doctor was also surprised to find a patient so young worried about his PSA. When I explained our crisis with Karen and my newfound belief in preventative maintenance, though, he saw no reason to discourage me. "After what you two have been through, this role reversal should give you both a new perspective."

Now came his explanation for the blood work. "The PSA records the level of cellular activity we need to monitor. If it reads at a certain level, a biopsy of the prostate is necessary. If anything unusual turns up during examination, this too can indicate the need for a biopsy to provide further information. I don't believe this will happen in your case, because of your age. But it is not too early to be careful, considering all you've told me."

All this was reassuring to me. Apparently my family history wasn't as alarming as I had assumed. Furthermore, when you reach your forties, it's a rare pleasure to hear that you are a little too young for *anything*. Maybe my intensive research into cancer had stampeded me into a doctor's office ahead of time. Karen, warming up to her role as supportive spouse, accepted the reassurance and relaxed a bit.

An examination followed, which was awkwardly painless but will best be left to the reader's imagination. Then the doctor announced, "You will be having a biopsy." Both of us jolted back upright. "I have felt an abnormal enlargement in the gland. I suspect it is merely a nodule. But the only way to be sure is to do a biopsy."

Both of us must have simultaneously thought, "Here we go again." I fought off a flurry of panicky notions and struggled to appear calm and businesslike. I knew that Karen needed the assurance of my strength, and then I briefly thought, "So this is what it's like to be the patient in a relationship." Meanwhile, Karen felt her first frustrations as the concerned bystander.

Despite my questions and speculations, the doctor insisted on assuring us that he believed my lump was merely a harmless nodule. "This procedure is simply a precaution," he told us both. "It's the only way to be sure you are all right."

We drove home that night over familiar roads and our conversation was a replay of many we have had in recent months. We discussed appointment dates and preferred clinics; we considered carefully who should be told and what should be said. Lawson Memorial Hospital was again chosen, since we were satisfied with Karen's radiation treatment so far. Karen comforted me with positive thoughts and living support; she knew exactly the emotions I was now exploring.

Over the next couple of weeks, we walked in each other's shoes as patient and supportive spouse. Karen discovered new dimensions in worrying, beyond those she felt in her own case. She began to dwell on the worst scenarios, just like I had in her case. But I felt like I was in control of the situation and enjoyed the luxury of reassuring her.

"You're right," she admitted. "It's easier to be the patient."

I had to admit that both roles have their disadvantages. But now I was the one saying that everything would be all right.

The doctor was right, and the biopsy proved it. A harmless nodule was all it turned out to be. So it was time to put that worry out of our minds and move on. We both still had Karen's treatment to endure. But this episode helped both of us understand the other's perspective. And once again, we felt the relief that comes from preventative care and early detection.

Karen wanted to do something for the staff at Lawson Memorial to let them know how much we appreciated their professionalism and consideration. I had an idea. "You know, one day while you were receiving your treatments, the technicians and I were talking about food. Imagine that. Well, she didn't seem too enthusiastic about cooking."

"Then why don't you make some of your famous caramel popcorn and bring it in for the girls to snack on?" I thought this was a great idea. It doesn't take much encouragement to get me to make popcorn. Our relations with the medical field had certainly improved.

One day in October while driving out in the country, I happened to be listening to a local radio station talk show when the topic of breast cancer came up. October was 'Breast Cancer Awareness' month and they listed some of the fund-raising activities going on in our community. Then they discussed some new and innovative procedures in breast cancer research. It seemed as if our life was now scripted for radio. I was very interested in hearing what they had to say. The announcer asked listeners to call in with their stories or any question regarding breast cancer and the treatments available.

"Our guest on the program this morning is the Director of the Waller **Cancer** Center in Louisville." I almost drove off the road. I knew right away that I had to call in and tell him our story about the way we were treated. I immediately raced toward home at an excessive speed, on a mission. This was my one big chance to go to the top with our story, on the radio before one hundred thousand listeners. What a great opportunity!

I needed to make this call from home so I wouldn't be interrupted. I'd probably be kept on hold for several minutes and I didn't want to let anything at work interfere with this opportunity.

As soon as I got home I dialed the number and surprisingly got right through. The call screener asked me for my comment and wanted to know if I wanted to be on the air. "I sure do." Within about thirty seconds, I was on the air.

"My wife and I have gone through two surgeries and we are currently in the process of taking radiation," I proclaimed to the world in general. "I believe it is important for cancer patients and their caregivers to battle the effects of cancer together. It is very important for the spouse and family to be included as much as possible. Spouses and family members suffer through this ordeal along with the patient."

The host of the program and the director of the Waller Center naturally agreed. The director explained in some detail how important it was for the families to be involved with the patient and how important their physical and emotional support was to the patient's recovery.

Now I had what I wanted. I had the director on record. "Well, then, let me tell you about my experience at your center." I went into as much detail as I could. To my surprise, I was allowed to speak my mind. And believe me, I unloaded. By the time I was finished he knew my displeasure with his center and its "policy." The listening audience learned that we received no cooperation from his center and instead endured official resistance in this matter, which the director had just said was vital to the patient's recovery. I emphasized that we had since moved and were now taking treatments across the river at Lawson Memorial.

I didn't get much further than that when he interrupted me: "I think we need to talk off the air." He wanted me to call him that afternoon so we could talk in further detail. I asked for his phone number and then got off the air. In a follow-up comment, the host stated how important she felt it was for families to be involved. I got what I wanted: my side of the story presented to the person in charge.

We played telephone tag a couple of times throughout the afternoon and finally connected about five o'clock. I got quickly to the point, recapping our side of the struggle at the Waller Center in extensive detail. I spoke for about thirty minutes. He only interrupted me on two occasions and when I finished I hoped for a rebuttal on his part. All I got was, "I'll look into it and call you back."

I'm still waiting—the call never came. I guess I was a little naïve to think I would get an answer. At least I was able to vent my frustration with his center to him and the listening audience of our local station. My testimony against this center had come just after the director had expressed his commitment to family involvement. He must have felt uncomfortable about this. Who knows? Maybe that changeable hospital policy changed again as the result of all this.

We met again with Dr. Carlisle for our weekly appointment and told him everything was going great. The technicians were being very cordial and understanding toward our preferences. I wanted to know, out of concern and curiosity, when Karen would begin turning red from the radiation. Dr. Carlisle stated that radiation is accumulative and she would be redder in the last several days of the treatments than she was now.

Each day we went to radiation helped us settle into a routine. My nervous feelings were still there, but I was adjusting better than before. Being the first patient of the day was a great convenience to us. We were in before most people were starting the workday and out in time to begin ours.

As we were winding up the treatments, I found myself counting down the days. Karen's vase of flowers was filling up nicely once again and the one at school was dwindling down each day. We met with Dr. Carlisle a couple of days before we finished the treatments and he said everything was going well. Karen had just now started turning red and becoming pretty tender. Dr. Carlisle assured us she would be just fine and the tenderness would be getting better a couple of days after the treatments ended.

On our last day of radiation, Karen received a graduation certificate signifying the end of treatments. She had passed and was now a cancer survivor. We thanked the girls who had worked so well with us and told them how much we appreciated them.

Over the next several days, the tenderness left her breast and the skin color returned to normal. Her stamina remained somewhat sluggish throughout the next couple of months. But her embattled spirit regained strength quickly.

We are now six months past our last treatment. Karen just had her baseline mammogram again and everything was perfect. We've met with the surgeon a couple of times since then and will do so for the next year and a half. He expects no problems. Our long ordeal is now almost over. Because Karen was taking tomoxifen, Dr. Pokorny suggested that she see her gynecologist to discuss some of the associated risk. The main risk is an increase in the chance of uterine cancer. Dr. Pokorny wanted Karen to discuss ways in which she can monitor and test for uterine cancer.

◆   ◆   ◆

I have tried to tell our story by writing this book. It has been very important for me to be involved with my wife each step of the way, including the documentation of our hopes and worries, our struggles and triumphs, and the relief of recovery. I hope by reading this you will be encouraged to take a similar role if the situation arises.

Every person reacts to cancer in a different way. Some people avoid the situation and refuse to talk about it. Others believe in supporting the patient, but choose to stay out of the way. We felt it was important for us to be fully involved, not only to be present at each step of the way, but also to share active roles resisting the disease. The two of us together just might figure out what the doctors were actually saying.

Together we researched this cancer and discussed the best ways to battle it.

At times this cancer came between us and made it difficult to go on. Like an unwanted stranger in the house, it strained the long-standing ease of our relationship. Both of us needed and received the support of our family and friends. Naturally, as survivors, we have become staunch advocates of preventative cancer screenings, and have encouraged several close friends to have their first mammogram. Naturally, we have recommended a few doctors and have also told them who to stay away from.

Cancer is a disease that not only invades the body: it also invades a relationship, family and lifestyle. Emotionally, the recovery period depends on how you approach the problem. Even though it took me a very long time to accept this threat, I feel better by doing so. Has it been hard? Extremely! Did our relationship grow because of it? I know it did and I know I'm a much better person because of it. I now know what other people go through and I feel somewhat qualified to make suggestions to them. I've learned now that until you've been through something like this, you really have no clue how difficult it is.

If I had any advice to give, it would be to get routine checkups and to listen to your doctors. Medicine has advanced so much in the last several years. What is a routine treatment today will be outdated in just a few years—what was once thought impossible is now coming quickly into sight. The quality of your life can be improved with early detection. There are many tests that can be taken to detect cancer and some of them are as simple as a blood test or x-ray. Don't be afraid to have these tests run because of what you might discover. The undiscovered truth is much more dangerous. Early detection is everything! The chances of survival skyrocket when cancer is discovered early. It is your life and you alone have the responsibility to take care of it. You're not a cat with nine lives, so make the most of the one you have.

If cancer is discovered, then something must be done. Throughout this book I have tried to convince the reader how important it is to get involved. As spouse or offspring, family member or friend, be there for the patient and support them in every way you can.

When talking with the doctors, ask questions. Don't let them rush you through a session, or feel intimidated because you don't understand. No question is a dumb question if you don't know the answer. Just remember they are working for you. You have employed them. You and your insurance company pay their bills. Don't hesitate to ask a question. Don't let them walk out of your room until all of your questions are answered. I encourage you to write questions down ahead of time so you won't be distracted and forget something. Come to the office prepared with a notebook or tape recorder in order to get everything recorded accurately. We all know that sometimes two people hear the same thing differently. If you are unsure of an answer you were given, ask them to provide you with some documentation supporting their conclusion. This can include anything from research material to magazine articles. Don't be afraid to follow up with the doctors after you have left their office. Some of your questions could be directed to nurses as well. They can be a great source of information.

My mother gave me one of our best sources of information. When my father had prostrate cancer about five years ago, she heard a public service announcement from the American Cancer Society encouraging people to call them at 1-800-ForCancer. When you call this number, they ask you what type of cancer you are dealing with. Within a couple of days you will have numerous easy-to-read booklets that contain several drawings and sample questions to ask your doctor. All of this material is free. It is mailed to your house. What could be easier? When we went to the doctor I even took this material with me. By reviewing this material before we met with the doctor, we were better prepared to understand just exactly what he was saying. This gave us greater insight into what was going to happen next and allowed us to actually have a lengthy, useful and mutually understood conversation with the doctor.

This has been our story. Did we do everything exactly right? No. There were numerous things we could have done differently. But our priority was sound. We both needed each other, and needed to be needed by the other. This became paramount to us, to share the burden in order to help the other and alleviate our own strain. I cannot imagine going through something like this on your own. With God's help, we won't have to again.

Just remember that early detection is everything. Don't gamble with your life because you're afraid of what you might find. It is the unknown threat, the unnamed stranger in your house, that produces the greatest fear. Facing the intruder together, as a team, you stand a better chance of chasing him away. Those improved odds might make all the difference.

0-595-22630-2

www.ingramcontent.com/pod-product-compliance
Lightning Source LLC
Chambersburg PA
CBHW020239290526
45784CB00003B/1033